SO YOU'VE HAD A STROKE

A survivors' guide to life after stroke

WILL DAVISON

Copyright © Will Davison 2017

All right reserved

The moral right of the author has been asserted

www.willdavison.info

CONTENTS

INTRODUCTION 1

JO ELLIOTT 4

BRENDAN KEHOE 21

MAUREEN (MO) CLARK 35

WILL STAMMERS 60

HEATHER LAWRENCE 74

JOHN DAVIS 100

COLIN McDERMOTT 114

DAVE COTTRELL 125

CHARLES SPENCER 138

ELIZABETH ASHMORE 157

AFTERWORD: WILL DAVISON 170

ACKNOWLEDGEMENTS 185

INTRODUCTION

Strokes don't happen; that's what I assumed. In fact I never thought about it at all. Sixty years of my life were spent in innocence. Yet according to the Stroke Association, stroke happens every three minutes and twenty seven seconds in the UK, to all ages and genders. That's one hundred and fifty two thousand times a year!

When I proposed the idea of a book on Stroke Survivors most people were very encouraging. They told me it was an interesting project and would serve as a source for many people who needed to know that there is life after stroke.

I was stunned, however, by one reaction. 'Boring', he said, with all the authority of the uninitiated. I had no instant response to this assessment, but since then, with the benefit of hindsight, I realize that the 'mot d'escalier', as the French have it – the killer response - would have been to come back with the one pertinent fact: This is my reality.

I have lived the last twelve years of my life, after two strokes, slowly recovering from physical impairment – limb paralysis, loss of speech and handwriting ability (thank goodness for the keyboard). It is also the reality of Colin, my cousin Ros's husband. They are featured in this book as one of the eleven stories of stroke survival; my own included. It has been a pleasure to talk to them all – diverse and different as they are. I trust the reader will find them interesting, insightful, uplifting and not at all boring.

Collecting the stories has been a personal adventure and has helped me understand my new stroke self. Travelling around the country to interview – by car or train - has even given me confidence to be less cautious about what I can achieve.

Make no mistake; stroke survivors are different from their former selves. Some welcome the changes that have taken place in them. All are aware of the weariness caused by stroke. Some have virtually no physical impairment; others are very much more seriously affected.

The most exciting finding (for me at least) is the discovery of the notion that brain plasticity is paramount. Given time stroke survivors find that there is hope, that the brain recovers and new routes within it are forged. The spectacular brain finds a way to reroute and restore function. I'm sure this is something we are to discover more about over the forthcoming years, and I recommend Prof. Charlie Stagg's work at Oxford University and viewing her inspiring video lecture on the subject*.

When I asked for 'advice to a new stroke survivor', almost everyone I talked to said, 'Don't give up'. When you feel isolated, frightened and alone with your new stroke condition, don't be put off by medical professionals, carers and loved ones, and even, sad to say, some stroke charity workers, who see us as poor souls with scant hope but who validate their money gathering.

Don't buy any of that. My feeling is that stroke happens for a reason in your life. It's not 'bad luck' or your life being cruel. Look on it as an experience that will do so much for you and those around you. Perhaps difficult to accept but something I truly believe.

Finally I want to thank all my Stroke Survivor interviewees for their honesty and openness in sharing their stories with me. I also want to thank my wife Annie who has unfailingly encouraged me, not only during my own strokes but also in the writing of this book. Wonderfully she transcribed all the interviews for me.

Will Davison

Prof Charlie Stagg's (Senior Research Fellow at St Edmund Hall, Oxford) Teddy Talk video on Brain Plasticity is available at:

https://www.seh-ox-ac.uk/about-college/talks-v-chapel

JO ELLIOTT

As I became more deeply aware of stroke I assumed, erroneously as it happens, that stroke only affected older men. Much later I began a search for women stroke survivors and fortunately Jo Elliott got in touch. She is now forty-five and had her stroke two years ago on holiday.

We have much in common. Both of us had strokes in France and were treated in a French hospital, where care is very good indeed; and in fact most hospitals are modern and in excellent condition. My local GP in France told me after my stroke that care in France is first class but the French now can't afford it! (remind you of anywhere?)

Jo Elliott is a Registrar of Births, Deaths and Marriages. Here is her story:

Two years ago I was a mum with three children, now twenty-one, eighteen and fifteen. I was fit. I worked as a Registrar for births deaths and marriages, three days a week. I also did at least a couple of weekends a month of ceremonies. I was outgoing and quite chatty. I cared what I looked like. I quite liked to wear high heels. I was a keen gardener, an avid shopper and life was quite full. I had friends that we would entertain either for weekends or dinner parties. And also I was quite house-proud. Life was quite full really.

When I had my stroke, two years ago, I was on holiday in France. We'd travelled down through France on the Friday. Because I had slightly older children I would take turns where I would sit in the car, so I didn't always have my legs right out in front of me as you do if you're sitting in the front of the car.

I had my stroke on the Monday morning first thing. I bent down to pick up the top of the barbecue grill, and as I was carrying it back inside I felt my leg give way. I felt a bit weird, nothing painful. I sat down on the nearest chair and immediately started shaking all over and couldn't stop. I felt so weird I said to my family 'I'm going to sit down on my bed'. Again I couldn't stop shaking, but at that stage my eye had begun to droop and also my mouth began to droop as well. My husband thought I must be having an epileptic fit or a stroke.

Once we had decided I needed medical attention I realised I couldn't walk when I got up to go to hospital. So my husband and my son carried me to the car. Unfortunately we didn't know the equivalent of dialling 999 so my daughter, with a satnav, had to find the nearest hospital. At that point we realised we were only four kilometres away from a hospital.

I feel tremendous guilt that the children had to be there. As I was having the stroke my children were just looking at me. I was having to apologise and say 'I'm really sorry, I don't know what's going on'. I feel really guilty that I put them through the whole event and the aftermath of it all. I think as a mother you always put your children before you, and I think that's something I will carry with me to the grave.

I must point out that I'm not overweight. I don't smoke. I drink, but not to excess – I'll have a little wine at weekends. I didn't have high cholesterol or high blood pressure; I had no risk factors.

When I got to the hospital, again it was very frightening because I didn't know what was happening. I was trying to normalise things, as with the drive to the hospital. I was pointing out, 'oh look at that lovely mansion over there', to the children. But obviously I didn't realise that my speech had already gone and they couldn't understand what I was saying. And also my vision had gone; I was getting a lot of double vision.

When we got to the hospital they couldn't get me out of the car. They managed to get a chair to wheel me in; I think just an office chair on wheels; very weird. But because of the language barrier we sat in the equivalent of A & E, and my husband after about five minutes managed to get us seen. They ran us through to the emergency bit very quickly. One funny thing, when I was being initially assessed my husband was told to 'pick the pockets' of the wife! My husband took all my rings off as I was still violently shaking.

Then I was taken into their main assessment area; very quickly they must have realised I'd had a stroke, so I was sent for an MRI. Obviously I was very frightened. You have to be very still, and it's also quite noisy. At that point, when I came back to my assessment room they told me I'd had a stroke. I was incredibly surprised. I was still shaking and couldn't even hold a glass of water; it would pour all over me.

I stayed in the assessment room for a couple of hours while my husband was liaising with the staff. Although we were quite near a big town they didn't have a good stroke unit, so they said they would transfer me to Toulon where they did have a specialised stroke unit. In order to do that my husband was asked for two hundred and fifty euros in cash, to pay a private ambulance driver to transfer me. I don't know if that's normal in France, but fortunately it was the beginning of our holiday and I happened to have a purse full of cash, which somebody had thought to bring. Had it been the end of the holiday we might not have had that.

I was then sent down to Toulon separately, I was on my own. I found that frightening. I was in and out of consciousness, and because I had tried to drink so much I was also desperate for the loo, and trying desperately not to lose my dignity and wet myself. I remember lying in the ambulance thinking I needed the loo, and when I arrived at the hospital I went straight to be assessed.

At that point my husband arrived. He didn't really know where he was aiming for; and then had to go through lots of information points to find the ward where I was and found me. That's when my care began. He was told that because the four hours had elapsed they couldn't do the thrombolysis clot busting treatment. They hadn't mentioned it at all to my husband at the previous hospital.

I saw my family maybe for half an hour, and then they were removed. I was in intensive care, and lay flat on my back for the next forty-eight hours. I did feel extremely alone and extremely frightened. I realised something bad was happening; I don't think I fully understood it at the time. So I just said to my husband, 'I am going to be okay aren't I?' and he promised to talk through with me everything they said to him. Not to have him say 'oh of course you will, it's fine', I thought, gosh I've got to dig really really deep here. And I think that was a turning point to help my recovery and everything else. I thought, this is actual life here and you don't get a second chance.

The care I got was exceptional in terms of nursing; one particular staff member was very kind, Celine - though I felt slightly embarrassed because I was just a tourist. They started raising me after the first forty-eight hours, by varying degrees. I'd had a brain stem stroke, a left Pontine Infarct, which had affected all of my right side, I couldn't use my arm or leg, and my face still drooping. The shaking did stop. I think now it's the brain sending out all sorts of signals and the body going haywire.

They got me out of bed quite quickly but all I could do was stand on my left leg. Obviously I couldn't do anything. I had to have a catheter to start off with but after that I had to get staff members to help me go to the loo. I couldn't get myself off the toilet; things were that bad initially. They were also giving me injections in my tummy; extra clot busting. If I travelled now over four hours in a plane I'd have to have that.

To give blood there you have to have a signature, and I realised I couldn't write. Nobody warned me about that. And as a registrar of births, deaths and marriages, that's what I did. At that point I thought, am I ever going to be able to work again, do my job? That was very worrying at the time.

Because of the language barrier they couldn't explain exactly what was happening. In France they wheel you to whichever consultant you're seeing and leave you in the corridor to wait. It was frightening because I wasn't aware of where I was going or what I was doing. Also the lack of family in the first few days was difficult because their visits were extremely limited. They had to travel an hour each way and they did that every day, and they would see me when hours of visiting were appropriate.

It was difficult watching my children cry, and also my youngest son, who was thirteen, withdrew into himself. He wouldn't speak to anyone, his dad. It wasn't until I came home and was beginning to get better at home that he started to return to his normal personality. He read a lot and his way of coping was to shut down.

I was transferred directly from intensive care to a side room on my own, thanks to the insistence of the lovely nurse Celine. My family were really good at that point; they would come at 12 o'clock when visiting started and they would stay with me until 8 pm in the evening. And basically I progressed and by the time I left the hospital I was able to walk with a frame - not very well; I was shuffling.

And my husband started taking on the duties that I think the nursing staff would have done. If I wanted to wash my hair, I would walk with the frame to the bathroom and he would wash my hair for me, and generally care for me. The staff were quite happy and accommodating about that; one less person to think about.

The tinnitus was really quite bad, which I still have. It's lessened and if I'm in conversation I don't really notice it, but if I'm not talking I can hear it. But I've been incredibly fortunate because I wanted to be repatriated back to England as early as I could and we managed to do that after ten days. Fortunately the insurance we had taken out for the holiday, everything was covered, so I was repatriated with my daughter and a nurse. The three of us flew back to Britain and down to Southampton hospital.

What was incredibly good of my husband was he asked the staff at Toulon – who he was very impressed by – if he could have a CD of all the tests and results that I could pass on to the hospital in the UK. I think that was crucial because I was determined to go home as soon as I got to the hospital; as much as anything I wanted some normality back for my children. The hardest thing is being so out of control.

Back home, the standard of the hospital was awful, compared to what I'd had in France. Being on a ward with about five ladies, all seventy plus, as a forty-five year old woman I just wanted to go home and get back to normality. What was interesting was that when I got to Southampton I could walk with a frame, but the very next morning I told the nurse I needed to go to the loo and could I have a frame and she said 'take my arm, I'm sure you can'. And although I was shuffling along I managed to do it and I was so keen to leave that I asked if I could go home. I ended up only having one night there.

One of the hardest things, being fit, I couldn't understand why it had happened. And the doctor did say only a third of stroke survivors know why it has happened. I had to do some tests to see if I was going to be okay on my own with the family. Like I had to go downstairs and buy something, then walk back up to the ward, to make sure I wasn't confused. I was doing little fairy steps, and because of balance issues I was struggling a lot. Twelve hours before I wouldn't have been able to get in the car, but it shows you how remarkable the brain is when it does put things back into place.

The consultant was very good and got me a care team to look after me at home. When I got home we were left for the night and then in the morning the Early Supported Discharge Team came out. The main problems were my speech and my arm. I was having increasing problems with my arm because I couldn't do any cooking; had no control to stir. In France I'd found it difficult to feed myself. Everything became difficult because I was right handed, but the team were fantastic.

For the next four weeks they did occupational therapy, speech therapy, and physio, which was mainly to increase my gait. I could walk to the local lamppost, about a hundred yards. My daughter had had her A level results and my son his GCSE results. I was in my own bubble of recovery and although I was pleased for them I think it didn't quite have the effect it would have had without the stroke. Nothing was really getting through to me.

But I didn't want to miss my daughter going off to university. I'd had the stroke on 28 July, and this was now the end of August and we needed to get everything ready. I had fierce fatigue but I didn't want to miss out on trips to Ikea and things. That's where the wheelchair came in useful. I did find the stimulus of being out and about, although it tired me out incredibly.

My stroke affected me so much in the first few weeks that my daughter offered to put her university back a year to be my full time carer, but the curve when I started healing was at such a dramatic rate, she didn't need to do that. I think my determination really got me through. It took a tremendous toll on my husband Howard. He had had to think through the repatriation.

Because he was a partner in a small surveying firm there was no opportunity to have compassionate leave, as the work had to be done. He had to work around his job and me for the first few weeks until we finally reached some normality. He hardly slept during that time.

I was so determined my stroke wasn't going to take my job away from me and that was what devastated me at the time; am I going to give up a job that I love. I started teaching myself to write again. It took about three months, and funnily enough my writing has come back exactly the same, though not as neat as it was, and sometimes I find I leave letters out, so the messages aren't getting down to my hand quickly enough.

One of my friends, a practice nurse, suggested at the beginning of September that I ask my consultant to give me a Bubble Echocardiogram to see if I might have a hole in the heart. She said that one of the things that could have happened, if I'd had a DVT (deep vein thrombosis) going down to the South of France, it could have travelled to my brain. It turned out that I did have a hole in the heart, and I've now had that closed. To have that reason helped put my mind at rest. I'm now on blood thinners and statins.

Being on long-term sick leave is quite lonely, isolating. At that time I didn't know anyone else who'd had a stroke at my age, so

I felt very different. Also, I didn't know how to behave. I was treating it like a bad case of flu in a way; I will get better. I lost confidence and put on a lot of weight because I was sedentary. Although I could walk again my stamina was hit, so I would use the wheelchair for longer journeys.

My recovery has been brilliant, but it was really challenging at times. I was getting very fatigued, and that has been my Achilles heel. But I'm good at time managing now. I know what I can do and what my body can go through. I have an iPhone. I use the calendar on that, and I build in rest days. At first I had to build in quite a lot of sleep, but then you don't want to give into it as well. So there's a little bit of fighting against your body.

My family have been so sympathetic, so supportive. I cannot fault them; my husband Howard especially, because a stroke affects the whole family. I had to develop a good sense of humour because in a way we're quite a tight family and we get endless banter. My way of coping because of the guilt was to become the class clown, trying to bring fun into the house; one of my coping strategies with the children. One of the benefits, my middle son gets me more than the other two. I don't think our relationship would have developed in the way it has had I not had the stroke.

When I was on sick leave I was really determined to get back to normal. As a lady of working age I wanted to get back to normality. At that stage I don't think I realised I'd never be able to get back to normal properly. I think when you're in a position where 'that could be it', it changes you. I now look at every day my glass half full. I look on the positives of each new day rather than dwelling on little insignificant things that could be negative: it's a waste of energy asking 'why me'. I think that determination of character really helped with my recovery. Also I've been quite driven and determined.

But I should point out there isn't enough advice given to general practitioners about strokes and this is a key problem for me. I think there's a general lack of understanding. I was the youngest stroke survivor that my doctor had had, and although she was fantastic to my husband when we were in France, talking him through procedures and medication, when I came back I felt she was a little bit out of her depth with me. I felt there was not enough knowledge about younger stroke survivors and what you can expect from their recovery; hence she pushed me back to work too early.

I went back to work after Christmas, but in hindsight I would have stayed off work much longer. I wouldn't have pushed myself too early, which I did. I completely relapsed. What should have been a phased return of six weeks back to what I was doing – three full days – 8.30am-4.30pm. We realised within three weeks there was no way I could do this. I had no idea how tired I would get. Just travelling to work and back was enough.

I ended up being really upset that I couldn't do it and my GP said 'she can't do more than four hours, ideally with a day between'. Work was good in that they offered to give me a permanent contract where I would be working two days, five hours a day for six months: April to September of that first year back – 2015. I worked back office so I wasn't in front of customers, but although I found I didn't have a problem with my memory or knowledge, I had a problem putting it altogether. The whole multi-tasking aspect was quite hard. When they tried to put me back to customer facing I was making mistakes daily. I couldn't keep up, and I found the 'customer led' emotion around a topic very draining.

Subsequently I spoke to my manager about leaving, and at that point they spoke about giving me a new role, not customer facing, with a permanent but reduced contract. Now I only work two days a week from 10am-3pm. It took a lot of heartache to get there. I also took neuro-psychology testing, which demonstrated that I was having high-level cognitive issues and that if I was tired I needed to build in breaks. That was quite helpful.

There is a pressure to get me back to doing ceremonies but they tire me out enormously, and I have the constant role of trying to educate my employer, as I look fine but there are challenging issues they can't see that they are trying to understand. But if I hadn't gone back to my job and I was at home 24/7, I think I would have begun to get a bit depressed. I feel fortunate that I'm able to do part of my job. I'm alive and I can do these things.

I considered myself always to be a nice person but I think now I have more empathy, not only with people with disability but with people generally. I have the patience to understand whatever anybody is going through. I do think the stroke is negative; I didn't wish for it to happen, but it has happened. And it's important and fundamental to me to be able to turn a negative into a positive, and that's where Different Strokes comes in.

It was incredibly beneficial to me to ring their head office and get the information when I first had my stroke. I had the number given to me by one of the therapists who came round and whose husband had had a stroke as well – at a younger age. I was nervous of going to any support groups because I was being very under confident, but eventually before Christmas I thought I'm going to do it and I've never looked back since.

I met people who still had difficulties. Some wheelchair users, some walking with sticks, some like me are fortunate that they have recovered to such a level. But the empathy and advice and signposting I've received from them, that I now can give to new members I really find invaluable and has enriched my life. I would say I was a busy woman. Now the stroke won't let me be busy like that but I'm more enriched by knowing the people I know now.

You can have sympathy from your family but you can't have empathy because they haven't been through the experience. And I think I would have found it much harder not having gone to a group that has that empathy. It's like having a second family in a way.

Amongst my friends I'm worse off, but amongst stroke survivors I'm better off. That has helped. You have to accept and love the new you. I see people coming in now who don't like themselves, still comparing themselves to who they were. And there's no way you're going to get that old person back, as much as you might want to.

I'm the secretary now and I help run the group. I find ways of funding, do some work with head office – I've recently done a study of how Different Strokes had helped someone. So when

I'm not working I'm not just sitting at home; I can pick up things but in my own time.

I do find I can cope on an everyday basis as long as nothing comes in the way. My son was going to university this year, so I was faced with getting him ready. At the end of the day you're still a mother; you've got to step up. I was also doing ceremonies and working and it was all too much. Even if your brain is working that alone tires you out. So I did have another little relapse around September.

So we have to plan really well what we're doing, and adapt what you're expecting of yourself; change your philosophy. I have a cleaner. If I tried to clean the downstairs of the house my speech would go. If I don't need to do something I won't do it, so I can put all my energy into what I have to do.

I find concerts are too much stimulus for my head. I can drive but driving at night is too much for my brain. I haven't had people to stay or done dinner parties since my stroke. When I get tired my balance goes and my speech goes. But this is small fry for me compared to people having daily challenges, so I do count my blessings.

BRENDAN KEHOE

Brendan Kehoe is the charismatic chairman of 'Stroke Club UK'*, an independent club that holds bi-weekly meetings in Abingdon and Didcot. He is fifty-six and had his stroke five years ago. He firmly believes in stroke survivors supporting each other, as only they themselves can know and understand what other survivors are going through.

After an unfortunate experience with a national charity, Brendan, along with Gary Gill and others (all stroke survivors) set up 'Stroke Club UK', offering regular meetings locally. Here's his story:

I was born in Germany with Irish parents; they always take the Mick out of me in the local pub. I was an avid golfer, played a twelve handicap. I loved golf; I loved cooking; dinner parties, stuff like that. Really… I'd dance. Now my arm doesn't work. I've got a tendency to fall over a lot; got no balance on my left-hand side. So if I don't think about the way I turn, down I go. I've broken my ankle, broken ribs, broken my fingers, blacked my eye. Been a bit of a nightmare, but there I go.

I've been in the motor trade all my life really, in fact three weeks before my stroke I'd just started a new job. I was in hospital for five months, and in that five months they kept my job open, they paid me, hoping I would be back as a salesman for a company called Heathrow Truck Centre.

Three weeks and that was all I'd worked for them. But, having said that, I was hoping that I would get better, but at the Oxford Centre for Enablement – a place where, when you have a stroke, they try to get you back to being able to walk and move things, unfortunately my arm just wouldn't go. I actually broke my ribs in hospital! I fell over in hospital and on to a chair, and broke two ribs. So that put me back because I was unable to do any exercises at all for three weeks. But still, still in hospital.

Even things like card games are impossible now because only having one hand you can't hold the cards. It's just so difficult. Everything is so difficult these days.

The great thing is, the cognitive side of me is okay, apart from remembering some words, and my short-term memory. You know, I'll leave the house, get down the road, and then think why have I left the house? And I have to come back to the house, come back in, look around; 'oh, that's why I left the house', and go again.

Apart from that, being Chairman of Stroke Club UK, anything that needs to be done in Stroke Club I deal with. Unfortunately nearly all our members have suffered cognitive trouble, so it's almost impossible to get them to do anything, even though they all say, 'yes, I can do that', it doesn't actually get done.

The biggest bit for me is not that they forget; it's that they can't figure out how to do it. They know what they want to do but their brain won't allow them to do it. You can see them scratching their heads thinking, 'I know, I used to be able to do this, what have I got to do?' And then it's always excuses why they haven't done it, which for me is really frustrating because I'd rather them say 'no, I can't do it'. But unfortunately people aren't like that. They think they can still do things they can't do.

I knew one hundred per cent what was happening to me. I was in a pub, believe it or not, having lunch. I was working so I was drinking Coke. I'd met some friends of mine and we were discussing things. So I said, right, I'll get some drinks. I went to stand up and my leg wouldn't move. I'd been sitting on my leg, like it had gone to sleep and I went to stand up, then my arm started to feel funny. I said to a friend sitting next to me, 'listen carefully I'm going to stand up now, if I start to fall, sit me back on the chair. Just do as I say'. So I went to stand up. He grabbed me, sat me back on the chair, and I said 'phone 999, I'm having a stroke'. I knew I was. I just knew I was having a stroke.

I think it's lucky that the aneurism I had hit the part of the brain that allowed me to know what was going on. Because I think that made a difference as to how my recovery has been. Because if I hadn't known what I was doing I think it would have been a lot worse.

I was in hospital within twenty minutes. They gave me a brain scan immediately. They gave me an injection of something; I don't know what it was. That's when they told me that it was actually an aneurism that had gone to my brain.

I was told later by the Professor, that if the aneurism had gone to my heart it would have killed me. So he said you're quite lucky that it went to your brain, even though it's not luck, it's one of those things. It meant that once they started giving me the medication I wasn't going to worry that it was going to happen again. It meant I had to put up with what I've got.

I thought I was going to die, I thought, this is it. All that was going through my head. I've got three children and I was just thinking, what are the kids going to do? I just thought, oh my God what's going to happen to the children? But I mean, they're grown up, so I shouldn't have had to worry about them, but you always do. My older son was working in Watford, and he was the first person to the hospital. He came down the M40 at a hundred and twenty miles an hour! Bless him.

I honestly thought I was going to die, but the great thing for me is that that doesn't actually faze me, dying. If you die you die.

I've had a good life. I've had three fantastic kids; they've all done well at university. My younger son has just finished his university course now. He's already got a job at British Aerospace, engineering. Fantastic. The others are both schoolteachers; what else do you need? Their lives are sorted, so it doesn't really worry me now. Every day I have now is an extra day.

I'm very pleased to be alive. My daughter is getting married next year - Good Friday next year. When I was in the hospital my daughter came into the hospital and said to me, 'dad you're not allowed to die until you walk me down the aisle! Once you've done that, that's it!' I'll walk her down the aisle, yes. I really do struggle to walk but I'll be walking her down the aisle without a doubt.

My thoughts on a 'cure', is that one day I hope something in my brain will start to take over the bits that have been damaged. I'm always exercising. Whenever people see me I'm pulling my hands up, pushing them down, closing my hands up again. I don't want my hand to go into an unnatural position, which is something that happens with a lot of stroke people. I don't want that, so I keep lifting the fingers, making sure it doesn't go into a clenched fist.

My ankle has been swollen for four years and there's nothing they can do about it, they said it is just part of the stroke. The last three, four or five days it's stopped feeling swollen and so that gives me a great lift. I can say I'm getting better. And the good thing for me, is that I'm really positive about everything, so I'm thinking, yes, I'm getting there, I'm going to get better. Now, if in thirty years time I haven't got better, I'll keep thinking, today's the day I'm going to get better. I just keep doing that! It's a much better way of being than being negative.

In Stroke Club UK we want to make people smile and laugh. We really don't want people who are being negative. There was one guy who came to see us when we first started two years ago and we actually said to him, 'look if you're not going to be positive we don't want you to come to Stroke Club because we don't want you to put people down, we want people to be happy when they come here'.

We sit; some of us drink beer, others drink coffees. We always have a lunch when we're there. Everyone smiles and talks about what's going on. If anybody needs help with paperwork; if they've got any worries about anything they may need to do about benefits or whatever, then we'll give them the answers to it. We won't advise them, we'll just tell them how we dealt with it. We don't want to advise anybody to do anything because that's not what we're there for.

But we're there just to help each other really, so all the people that come are as positive as they can be anyway. We've got some there now – probably only one – who is so negative, but we're trying to get him out of that. He's in a wheelchair; he's always got his head down; he doesn't talk a lot, so we try to bolster him. If he comes into the meeting with his head down, by the time he leaves the meeting his head is up, and he's looking around and he's talking to people. So it is working. It's an uphill battle all the time, but the feeling of the good you're doing is much better than the feeling you might be doing something bad, so we just try every day to make people feel happy.

Regarding why it happened. I don't care because it has. The Stroke Association is a multi-million pound business, and they send people, university students to find why stroke happens and how they can stop it from happening. We're not interested in anything like that, because it's already happened to us. What we want to do is when someone has had a stroke, make them understand that they can improve. And if they can't get better they can at least have a life after stroke.

We've got one guy who, again, is in a wheelchair; an electric wheelchair; and he can't speak very well, and when he had his stroke his wife was almost suicidal because she just didn't know what to do, so it was dreadful. But for the last two years at Stroke Club, we've watched him go from someone who didn't want to do anything at all, to someone who at the Christmas Party got out of his wheelchair and was dancing. Well, not dancing, but out of his chair. And we'd just been to Weymouth – we take everyone to Weymouth every year – and he actually went ninepin bowling; sitting in the chair, but he did it. Now you can suddenly see him smiling and trying to interact with people, so it's a great thing.

Carers are everything to most stroke survivors. They don't mean anything to me personally because if I can't do it, then it's not going to happen. It's as simple as that! But I know: Paul, one of the guys, without his carer he'd be lost completely. His wife does absolutely everything for him. And there are quite a few of them like that. They need their carers there, they're so important.

Carers are a lifeline to a lot of people. Because the one thing I can remember vividly when I first had my stroke was how alone I felt. How lonely it was; a dreadful place to be. I'm lucky because I've got the children; I don't see them that often. As I said, my older son was working in Watford. He now lives in Dubai, so he's miles away. My daughter lives ten, fifteen miles away, and my other son has only just finished at Loughborough University. So they are not really close by, even though they'll phone all the time, ask 'how you doing, is everything okay?' You still feel, especially at night times, how lonely it could be.

Luckily now I've got a partner now, a girlfriend, who lives with me. And that makes all the difference. It's great to have someone there. She knew exactly my condition before we got together. I think it's the same as anybody, you think when you're like this 'that's it', you'll never get another girlfriend again. But she was actually married to a stroke survivor.

He's got the cat. He was going to have both cats but he couldn't cope with both of them, so I said you'd better bring one over here. She brings the cat over here and I find out I'm allergic to them: brilliant! Wheezing and sneezing, eyes running; typical! But I'm getting over that now, because I've always said, with things like allergies, if you face them eventually your body sorts them out and stops them from happening and it has been working. The wheezes are getting much better; I don't cough so much as I used to; my eyes don't run as much as they did; not so itchy, so it is working, slowly but surely.

I can drive. I can't walk around a shop because I get half way and I have to stop, and that's it then. If I use my leg too much it just stops working. I can't go anywhere. My foot drops; it just won't go anywhere at all. So I have to be really careful how far I will actually walk. I've got a travel buggy in the car, so if we're going anywhere I always use the buggy.

I can write. My right hand's fine. What I struggle with is I can't put my left hand out to hold the paper. That's the only reason I don't write much now. My arm doesn't work. I just can't get that better. Apparently; can't think what they're called; the things on your arm that hold, not the muscles, the other bits, are dead. If I try too much work with my arm it pulls the arm out of its socket because the muscles are still dead. I mustn't pull the arm out of its socket; have to be careful not to allow that to happen. And it aches all the time. No matter what I do with it, it's always got an ache, because the muscles are always trying to pull against the tendons.

I take Gabapentin; it's a muscle relaxant; the sort of thing they give people who have epilepsy. In the first instance they thought my arm had epilepsy, and I got a letter from the DVLA saying we're taking your driving licence off you because you've got epilepsy. And I said they reckon my arm might have epilepsy but I haven't. But they said no, the word epilepsy, means you can't drive.

I had to go to hospital to have an EEG, which is putting little steel discs over your head for them to come back to me to say it's not epilepsy, it was stasisity. So they didn't take my licence off me, which is a bit of luck because I don't know what I'd have done without that. I need to be able to drive, to get about. Especially running Stroke Club because we've got two areas:

Didcot and Abingdon, on alternate weeks, so I need to get between the two. I wouldn't be able to get anywhere without the use of a car.

If someone has already had a stroke my advice would be just please, please realise that your life is not over. It might be different but it's not over, and you need to get yourself to a stage where you can say, 'this has happened, this is how I am now, so let's start my life again the way I am.' But don't, please, think your life's over - because so many people do. Everything I've ever done before is past. The cooking, the dance, everything has now gone. I'm in a different place and I need to sort out what I'm doing now, so I see it completely differently now.

I still go on holiday. I've been to Dubai to see Liam a few times. Went over there to watch the golf. Hired a buggy while I was there, and because I was in a buggy I was allowed to go on the course with the players. So I was having a long chat to all the players. It was great. There is a young lad from Abingdon called Eddie Pepperell who plays on the European tour, and we all go there to watch him. So when we were over there the crowd is mostly from Abingdon because everyone goes over to see how he gets on. I've been to Portugal, Spain, Egypt, all after my stroke. Canary Islands. No, it's not going to stop me.

I have so many friends; it's incredible. When I first had my stroke I used to have real trouble with waterworks and I used to wee myself as regular as clockwork, and that is just so embarrassing, and you feel so low. But every one of my mates was always, 'hey, come on, don't worry about it; it's fine'. Everyone was the same.

Because of that, every single one of them were behind me and hence the reason why Stroke Club has done so well. All helped to fund it and look after everybody. So I've never had a problem. But I do know some of our members, their friends wouldn't talk to them any more. Just abandoned them. They have no idea why. Stopped phoning, stopped going round. Didn't know how to talk to them.

There are guys who go to Stroke Club now who can't speak properly, but it's I think it's really important that you engage with them. They might not be able to speak, but they still want you to speak to them, still want to be involved with you. Everyone gets spoken to, everybody. It's important.

I take one pill a day for my bowels; that just makes an incredible difference. Before I had to be within ten foot of a toilet just in case, because once I needed to go, I needed to go there and then. And now these pills are fantastic. Makes my life so much easier. Because I've always been open with everybody about what's going on, people know how I am. I'm very straightforward, and if I feel something I'll tell them that, and people like that. They like people to be straight with them and honest about what's happening.

Stroke is a dreadful, dreadful thing to happen to anybody. It annoys me more than anything when it happens to older people, because I was quite young, I was only fifties, very early fifties, so I am able to get over it a lot easier. People a bit older find it much more difficult to get over that first hurdle. It saddens me when I see people like that, it really does, but I'm not allowed to show that I'm sad. You have to show that you're happy. I take the Micky a lot out of them. I giggle a lot with them. And I know that makes them feel better, because they feel they are being treated as ordinary people.

The pubs that we've chosen as our venues, the reason why we've chosen them is because the people that run them understand exactly what we understand; everybody is treated the same way, as if they are ordinary human beings with a bit of an affliction. And it works every time. Whatever you do, just don't feel sad for someone who's had a stroke. Just accept that they've had one and help them get round it. Whatever it is they might need; whatever help they might need. That's the way to do it.

We'll be walking out somewhere and I'll say, hurry up will you, haven't got all day! Things like that: and they'll sort of laugh, or there's one guy, I said, 'do you want a race!' That's the kind of thing we do and because it's all about smiling, all about having fun, and spending the rest of your life with a smile on your face; not with a frown.

*www.strokeclubuk.org

MAUREEN (MO) CLARK

To say the least Maureen Clark is a live wire, in spirit anyway. Mo is probably one of the more physically impaired of all the stroke survivors I interviewed. I didn't need to ask questions. As soon as I switched on my recorder it all came bubbling out!

Mo has a series of carers throughout the day but her care is over-seen by her mother Verity. Verity is now 85 years old and was born in India. At the age of eight, she was sent to a prestigious boarding school in the foothills of the Himalayas. Verity is naturally concerned, as an older parent, for Maureen's long tem security. Both mother and daughter are delightfully strong characters, which is obvious when you meet them. They have asked that their names be changed.

Here is Mo's story:

I was a teacher. I used to work with visually impaired children; I used to teach blind children to read Braille; to work in families and schools and homes and things. I used to read Braille, not with my fingers but with my eyes. The theory is that you read with your dominant hand – invariably your right one – to the end of the line you are reading, and then the other hand... the second hand comes in handy because the beginning of the line you're reading, then down to the next line. It's like a Z. But children very rarely get to that by the stage I have them. It's a long process.

I did a degree in psychology, which I've been told on numerous occasions is not worth the paper it's written on: thank you very much! And then I wanted to change the world like most budding psychologists do. I did placements in schools and in hospitals; and I couldn't quite come to terms with adults somehow. Didn't have the patience with the adults, so thought with children at least there's a future to work on.

So I did my teacher training qualification. I left teacher training college in 1975 - the year there were something like two hundred unemployed teachers. I know it's difficult to tell by looking at me but I can't tell a story and play the piano at the same time. And God knows what teachers have to do these days, I can't. So I struggled to get a job.

Eventually, near where my parents lived, which was Northamptonshire, I got a job. I was a classroom assistant in an RNIB school for children with multiple difficulties. Of course they thought they were quids in having a qualified teacher, because it meant legally they could leave me with groups. It didn't matter what I did sadly. But at least I was able to learn things there, and gain from the experience.

Then I got a teaching job in a school in Leicester. To teach blind children you have to have an additional qualification, so I did that. And about that time computers were coming into their own - talking computers - and I found that quite interesting. Then I got a job in Bradford and rose to the dizzy heights of deputy head. At that time there were more special schools than there are now - there are lots of services that help children in mainstream. So I thought to myself: my ambition originally was to be head of a small school, and I more or less did that – I was acting head – so I thought I either stay in schools or I move into services and support work.

As luck would have it, I was living near Bradford at the time, there was a job going in Leeds in support services, so I applied for that and like an idiot I got it. So I moved into support services; trained to be an OFSTED inspector, which was horrible. Then in 2002, when the government were really coming down hard on local authorities and particularly big metropolitan city councils - which Leeds was at that time - we were inspected as an authority and we failed, or so they said. So we were outsourced to a private company.

They came in and did a thorough best value inspection, sort of a management thing, and where there had been two services: a support service for hearing children and a support service for visually impaired children: (I was head of support service for visually impaired children), the outcome of this supposed inspection was that they should combine the two and have one sensory service. Nobody ever told me why, but they said it was to become more efficient and effective. Huh! So there were all these reorganisations of jobs and things: people had to apply for their own jobs and stuff. There were two of us who applied for the head of support sensory service and with one girl who had been there for ten years, to one who had been there ten months, you know who's going to get the job. So the person who'd been there ten months got the job.

So I thought to myself, right, either I drink myself stupid, go and play on the M62, or I move. So I decided to move and there was a job here in Dorset. I thought, 'that's the job I've been doing, I can do it'. So I applied and hence I crossed the north-south divide and came to the south coast.

Then in 2011 it starts to go wrong. I was diagnosed with advanced bowel cancer. And that's when the rot started literally, and my mother sort of moved in then. I had an operation for the cancer. It had already spread to my liver, so I had an operation for that. I had one dose of chemotherapy, and the week after it finished, wham-bam, I had my stroke. That was 2012.

I think I was asleep in bed. Ultimately found myself on the floor. So I think I must have fallen out of bed, but I don't remember doing all these things. The only thing I can remember is I was in bed and my left arm was flopped over, and the arm couldn't feel anything. But I didn't think anything more about it. You don't at the time. I thought to myself, 'whose arm is that? It's not mine'. So I did the usual thing and I felt, 'oh yes, it is mine'. Still didn't think any more.

I was on the floor. I was trying to get up. I just kept sliding, because I couldn't do anything with this left leg and I wasn't strong enough to push myself up with the other one. Or didn't know the right techniques. So I called out. There was a friend with me at the time, which was lucky.

She called some other friends over and then the ambulance came. The ambulance driver did the usual: can you smile? Can you lift your arms? Can you do all this? None of which I could do. He said, 'I think you've had a stroke love'. So at the time you think, 'oh, all right, okay'. I was swiftly taken to the area hospital where I suppose I woke up at some time. They said, 'yes, you've had a stroke'. But even then it was… nothing, no explanations. You've had a stroke. So… nothing.

Since then I've got a weakness down my left side. And whilst I was in the area hospital, in a special unit, the physio there, I mean all they did was hoist me out of bed. I sat in a proper chair for a while to get my balance back, because they told me I'd lost my mid-line. Fortunately I know what that is, having learned with the blind children. It's a sort of saving reaction thing; that if you fall too far one way you automatically compensate. I'd lost that. But they kept using all these words I had no idea what they meant.

Because of my job and I knew about rehab, things like that, or where to go for help, I was at an advantage, because I certainly didn't get that much help in the first hospital. As I say, all the physios did... sometimes they'd come round, stand at the end of the bed, like a mumbling group of whatever, wise men, and they'd look at my left leg and go 'huh...still nothing?' And then the consultant would come and he'd say 'still nothing?' Yes, still nothing.

So then I was moved to the local Community Hospital, which is a sort of rehab hospital, and the team there were a bit more jolly; they were very friendly, and I remember a physio bounced in and said, 'what do you want to be able to do Maureen?' So I said I want to be able to get out of this bed and walk to that bathroom, and go to the loo by myself. 'Ooh... you won't be able to do that'.

Okay! And it was never a case that you might be able to do this. It was always 'ooh no'. You know, the same old story really. It was all fairly negative, focussing on what I couldn't do. I was very much left to myself to find out what I could do.

I was quite lucky because at the original hospital I got quite friendly with the chaplain there and he used to come along, and I'd tell him my tales of woe, and he'd say 'you want me to tell somebody that?' Go on then. So he'd tell people. Then the next thing they'd come along and say 'I hear you're not too happy with things'. I said 'well, no, would you be?' So at least in the Community Hospital I got out of bed and not just into a chair, but on to my feet. And for the first time I was able to do something albeit with a lot of help.

The one thing you want to do is go home, even though somebody might have said that reality should have kicked in and that it's going to be very different when you're home: there aren't nurses around at the press of a button. Nobody really said that, or made you face up to it, because your burning desire is to get home.

Anyway, I came home and my bedroom was the dining room. I had about six weeks of the community rehab team from the hospital: the physio, the OT (occupational therapist). The physio was good. She got me up walking and I had a frame thing. And I had carers come in. They still come in. Because I was still being hoisted I had carers in the morning, and then again at about ten o'clock, and then at lunchtime; then again at about four; then at about seven. So it was getting used to that: people coming into your home. But fortunately the girls that worked for the company were very good, very nice, and subsequently became friends. Yes, they are a good laugh, and they keep you going.

They keep me practising. I used to have to practise walking round downstairs and they'd walk behind me with my chair. They were very good. The OT sent a couple of his rehab workers. Now bearing in mind that I used to work with visually impaired children I know what rehab workers are and I know what good they can do, or what they should be able to do.

So these two beauties came – my mother will tell you her side of the story: she used to call them Hinge and Bracket – I mean, that's another thing... my mother came down when I was having my operations and she's stayed ever since, so that's a big thing; my mother moving in. And it's not a natural relationship. We're both fiercely independent. She's a self-confessed martinet, and she'll tell you this. Or she should do!

So these two beauties came to my home and asked me what would you like to be able to do? I said I'd still like to be able to some cooking. I used to enjoy cooking. So we went into the kitchen and they started to get things out, where upon my mother, bless her, came and told them what she thought of them. So they left and never came back! But what I really wanted them to be able to do was to come and give me tips, like 'people with one hand find it useful to do this'.

Now I've got gadgets. I know where to get them from, so I got them myself anyway. There's a little shop where you can go and get spiked boards and all this business. But if you can't see there are gadgets there are tips you can use to be able to do things, like 'don't make a cake that way, it's just asking for trouble. It's much easier, much quicker this way. It might not be a proper cake but it's a cake'. But no, none of that business, so a lot of it I had to find out for myself.

I've got a trolley for moving things around; otherwise I use my teeth! Most things have got teeth marks in them because I carry things in my mouth like a dog. If you ever get a letter with teeth marks in you'll know it'll be me! Coping is one of our saving graces really.

At the end of 2012 I retired from my work, because basically it was made clear that although I could still do management tasks, and appraisals, they said the things you can do is not the job we need. Having been on the other side of it you know exactly what that means. So I did the honourable thing and threw myself on my sword and took early retirement. I can't drive, or I couldn't then. I still can't. And I certainly couldn't go into people's homes and say I'll sit on the floor and play with children. I'd be stuck there for the rest of the day!

I remember early on asking the physio was there anything else that I could do, like more exercise, because I was slowly getting fatter and fatter, not doing too much exercise. She suggested swimming, so I used to go swimming at a local pool. Twice a week they have a higher rate of pool staff, and they have a hoist thing, so I used to go there with one of the carers. But the problem there was the water was very cold and it takes me a long time to get warm, and sometimes on a Monday I'd go swimming and I wasn't really warm until I went to bed again that night. So I gave that up.

I found out – again, all self-discovery really – about an exercise group for after stroke. So I started going to that. She's a sort of tough-love lady. It's great. She's been trained by the ARNI method, which is an American method. It's more about functional exercises: 'we're doing this because this might help you this way.' I go now twice a week and it's a good laugh and it's got me walking better. I walk without a stick.

Not that I can get up and walk wherever; it just means I can get myself out of trouble. So when I'm in here and my stick is in the kitchen and the trolley with the cups on has been brought in here and then taken out by mum absent-mindedly, I can get from here to there if I have to. That's sort of given me my independence back I think.

One of the things we do at this exercise group; exercise bikes. When I get on I try and do a kilometre. A lot of the time is keeping my balance. I've only got the one hand to hold on with, which is hard work, however hard you try, and even now I can't dress myself, which is very frustrating. I can't walk without the splint and I cannot put it on myself. It's like an octopus with velcro arms, so as soon as one goes one way, the other goes the other. But I have another type coming, which has taken nearly a year. Everything's slow, but they don't seem to realise that when they're being slow, it's missed opportunities for me, to maybe be able to move forward.

I was married before the stroke and we're on friendly terms. He does still visit, but my mother is my carer and it is frustrating - it is for me. I mean, she's parenting me: I don't need to be parented. I know I need help. I know there are things I can't do. But there are also things I wouldn't attempt to do if I didn't think I could do them. But my mother, because she's parenting me all the time, often jumps in and says 'no, you can't do that', which is very frustrating. We shout a lot; at least, I shout.

She's not been well either. Not that I've been able to do much. I'm an only child. It's always been just me. She's eighty-five. I mean, this isn't a real relationship. It's not normal for an eighty-five year old woman to be living with her sixty-two year old daughter and looking after her still. Whilst I used to live at home until I was eighteen, that was a long time ago and we were different people then. And going home at weekends is different. My dad was around. I'm a different person. I've got a very short fuse; I always have had but it's even shorter now.

I think the stroke has exacerbated that because I get very cross; cross with myself. I get cross about the situation, but there's nothing I can do about it. And people say, 'oh you're wonderful, you keep trying', and you feel like saying 'what choice is there?' You know it's not a choice to lie in bed all day and not work hard. Who in their right minds would not chose to struggle on manfully? I'm sure there are people who don't want to do it, but that's not me. I'm not going to let it beat me; that's for sure.

I'd say to someone who has newly had a stroke and just coming to terms, 'keep trying'. Accept that things will never ever, ever, ever, be the same again. You will never, ever, ever, be the person you were. But you'll be a different person. People in hospital would say 'don't worry, you'll get there'. I wanted to shout out 'where is there? How will I know when I'm there?' Other people would say 'the there is where you want it to be'. This isn't where I wanted to be, believe me. This wasn't on my bucket list.

You know, when I was a little girl and people said 'what do you want to do when you grow up?' it never entered my head to say 'I want to be a wheelchair user please.' But you are, so you have to get on with it. And it's just that... yes, you have to try and see the funny side of things; a laugh a day keeps the grumps away. I think that's what kept me going these many, many years.

I was very lucky; my friends have stuck with me, and come to see me, even though I'm far away. And I think as well, because we're all more or less the same age it's a bit of a wake-up call for your peers, as a fatal illness, or whatever, because it makes you think of yourself I think. I'm not selfish or anything but we had a reunion of old college people and I think they were all a bit dumbstruck, because in a way it could have been them. I don't think any one of them thought 'thank God it's her', because you don't think like that, but it could have been them.

And yes, the friend who was with me when I had my stroke, she comes down at least once a year. We used to go on holiday together, and I always said to myself I don't mind if my carers become friends, because that's nice. But I don't want my friends to become carers, because that's something different. So we still do things together. I'm trying to learn Italian. Not just because

I've read so much that being bi-lingual is good for the brain – good for the brain plasticity – but because it's this particular friend and we used to go to Italy quite a lot. The class comes here every Wednesday. It's good; good for a laugh.

So I'm trying to keep the body going and to keep the mind going. My short-term memory is appalling but my long-term memory is not too bad. My language didn't go, so I was lucky. I think I lost some mathematical abilities. I used to be good at Maths. I used to be able to think numbers. I find it difficult now; time doesn't necessarily mean anything, particularly these wretched digital clocks. Now is that 11.38, or is it 1, 13, 8? I have no idea which one is right or wrong. And, I ask my mother to distraction. And I've got a patch here - a blind spot - where I don't notice things. Not proper hemianopia, it's just if something is put down or I don't notice someone is actually physically doing something, I won't see it until I've had a good look. That's very common with strokes. I know that because of the job I did.

I tend to go away with my mother. For the first time this year I'm going away without my mother, but with one of the carers who has become a good friend, and another carer who left, but has remained a friend. We're going to London for the weekend. That'll be different.

I do slump in the afternoon. I think my enthusiasm is greater than my ability. You know, the mind is willing but the flesh is weak. I usually sit in here, in the front room, or nod off in a chair. I haven't gone upstairs to bed during the day for a long while. Let me think. I came out of hospital in the March. I think it was something like the following year, October, when I got the chair lift and I was able to get upstairs.

It's an odd tiredness at first. When I was in hospital I could only describe it as sheer exhaustion. You know, you close your eyes and the next minute you'd be asleep. It wasn't because you were tired or wanted to snooze. It was sheer exhaustion, just the effort of sitting up, or thinking and talking, and having a conversation, just wears you out.

Every year there's a thing called Step Out For Stroke, which is a walk basically, which I've done for a few years now. So I've walked a third of a mile in an hour. But at least I've done it. Everyone's been told 'oh you'll never do that, you'll never walk again'. But I suppose we're all different, you just don't know.

All that was ever said was that 'you've had a very dense stroke' and I didn't know what that meant. What does 'dense' mean? I think it means 'bad'. I think what they meant was that it was very big and bad. I don't think anybody told me what it was going to be like. I can't remember anybody telling me anything. I think it was perhaps only after reading things you begin to realise that's what's wrong is your brain; that takes a bit of getting used to as well. Yes, you're brain damaged actually, which is what you are. Because I'd look at my foot and think, well I've still got a foot, I've still got ten toes, why won't they work? People tell you, but you just hear perhaps every other word; you certainly don't put it together.

It's certainly a curved ball, because there are so many things that are stopped. Somewhere along the line I think I have lost myself. I don't know who I am any more. The person I used to be; I can't be any more. Or I try to be, as much as I can but it's the indignity of it, the dependency it causes, the loss of personal space and stuff like that. My ex-husband said 'you might look different, but you're the same person underneath'. I suppose that was quite telling. It was good.

I think it's given me a greater understanding into what I used to do. Because I know there are ways around things and you can adapt things but you end up changing it so much it's actually not what it was; the enjoyment factor's gone. I could go and do so and so, but having changed it all, perhaps it's not the same.

Most difficult; loss of independence; the humiliation – although I've got used to it - of someone having to take you to the toilet. I was so chuffed with myself the first time I managed to get out of the wheelchair and walk to the loo and come back. 'Ooh, look what I did!'

The loss of immediacy as well. You can't just sit down and think 'I know what I'll do. It's not raining. I'll walk down there and see if Fred's in.' But by the time you've got down there and Fred's not in, you've got to bloody well walk back again!

Verity says:

As a child, our last few years in India we were in boarding schools, all three of us, in the foothills of the Himalyas. I don't think my father could have cared less as long as he had his hunting, shooting and fishing. However we had a wonderful childhood in India - very different from growing up in England. When we had our daughter I decided that she would also have a good education. We paid for her schooling; she went to a convent school.

When we were coming to England my mother said, 'what you've got to do is finish your training' – I had decided to be a nurse. We came in 1948 when I was seventeen, trained at the Queen Elizabeth, Birmingham, met my future husband in 1949 and kept him waiting until '53! I made sure my mother never met my future husband before she went back to India, as she would have nipped a blossoming relationship in the bud! We had been together for fifty-eight years before he died at the age of eighty-three.

About June or July 2011 Mo told me she had been investigated for bowel cancer. And on her birthday she had the resection of bowel and two areas in the liver. So I came down; I was living in Northamptonshire. My brother joined me and we went to see her in hospital.

That was successfully removed. She also had two areas in her liver, which meant she had to go to Basingstoke. So I came back down and stayed here, and took her in to hospital, and visited her and brought her home when she was discharged.

That Christmas we went to Canada; we asked the doctors if it was okay and they said yes. She had 75 mgs of aspirin before we went, the usual thing if you're flying. We had a nice Christmas, came home, spent New Year here and I went back to my home to get my stuff, because I was going on a cruise. I didn't want to go on – I said I'd cancel it. She insisted I should go on the cruise.

She started her chemotherapy; and I think about two weeks after that, while I was on the high seas, I had a ship to shore phone call to say that she'd had a stroke. Fortunately we were coming into Tenerife the next day. Had we gone past that I would have had to wait until we got to New York, or Barbados, somewhere like that.

The officers on the ship were very good. They organised a flight and taxis and everything. My friend and I flew from Tenerife to Heathrow, and of course we were communicating with whoever was here, her friend Lyn. We got home about two in the morning. My brother was already here. By this time Maureen was in Southampton. So the next day we went there and I spoke to the consultant for the first time, and was told it was a bad stroke. Because they weren't going to operate on her to relieve any pressure – which is why I was asked to come home – she was sent back to her local hospital.

They were very good, very kind to her there, and looked after her very well. However, I think they gave up a little too soon. They used to get her up out of bed in the afternoons, and on the third day when I went to see her - they allowed me to spend a lot longer hours than I was supposed to - she was in bed. I asked the consultant why she hadn't been taken out of bed for this day, and he said the physios had decided that her leg was not going to make any improvements; I thought they'd given up on her.

I asked him if on the strength of just taking her out twice they could make that decision, and he said 'yes'. He said, 'don't worry we're not going to give up on her'. I confess I did badger him. So they kept her there and looked after her because she did have a tummy bug. I went home to Northamptonshire to sort out a few things and while I was there the consultant rang me to say they were moving her to her community hospital. I came back – the day she was moving – and she stayed there for a couple of months.

Mo asked the nurse practitioner when she was going home. The girl said she was being fast tracked, implying that the timing was crucial. Mo piped up and said 'does that mean I'm going to pop off in about ten days time?' 'Oh no', she says, 'it'll be a bit longer, about three months'. Now, we hadn't a clue about this.

Anyway, we swallowed that, and when I came home I phoned and spoke to all but one of the consultants, to see where this prognosis had come from. The long and the short of it was, none of those I spoke to said this was what they had said.

So we just accepted it, and of course she didn't pop off in three months time, as you can see. In March she came home to a hospital bed downstairs and had carers four times a day. She was hoisted in and out when necessary. She improved gradually and within six months we had a stair lift put in so she could sleep in her own bed. This made a tremendous difference to her mobility.

When we told one of the other consultants and the follow-up liaison nurse how we'd been told about the three months prognosis, they were flabbergasted. I said I still hadn't got to the bottom of where this had come from, because there was still one consultant I hadn't been able to chase up. I think it was because this particular surgeon was so flabbergasted, that we did get an appointment to see the consultant who reputedly made this remark. But when we spoke to him he said it was a case of Chinese whispers!

They were all very amazed with her progress, and when we saw the stroke consultant again, in about maybe six months, Maureen walked in with her tripod thing and he said that she had confounded them all. Now it is five years later and she's still going strong. So she's gone from strength to strength. We've had lots of to-ing and fro-ing to hospital for follow-ups. She has to maintain what she's got – it's not going to get any better – by keeping active.

What is it like being a carer? Well, I'm her mother for a start. And I'm also a nurse. It's a tie; it's changed my life. In the beginning I could only go up to my own home when someone was here; when one of her friends would come and stay with her. This meant I never had more than about six days, a week at the most, which was rare. And in the meantime my neighbour and my friend, were looking after my house, which wasn't fair to them. So in the end I decided I would sell the house. Last January I sold it, and so I'm here, homeless – that is, not a 'house owner'!

Maureen gets a bit frustrated, a bit paranoid sometimes with me. Occasionally I answer back, or else I just walk away. It's understandable. To a certain extent she might be able to manage without me, but there are certain things that she can't do without help; however much she would like to. To have got this far is an achievement. One thing Maureen has lost is her sense of time. I have to nag her to be ready in time if we have a deadline to keep. This is stressful for both of us.

You do have to change your outlook on life, and have to understand your limitations, I suppose. I have never let anything stop me. If I haven't got the strength in my arms I use my head, and my backside, and my knees. But now we have to ask for help if she falls. I can't lift her. Our neighbours came across a couple of times, but she very rarely falls now; but when she first started walking she fell a few times, and sent me flying as well. Fortunately I didn't get hurt, neither did she.

I sent her flying once. She'd been out in her wheelchair, and it's got a lever at the bottom that you pull out; it's got a sort of foot on it so that when you go up slopes it helps you to go up the pavement; it's on a sort of spring. So I was kneeling on the floor;

we were in the sitting room fortunately, and I pushed this in, but I wasn't strong enough to push it all the way, so it flew back up, hit me, I fell over, knocked her and she fell over, so the pair of us were on the floor! I phoned a friend of mine, only a little fella, and on his way up he passed another friend, six foot tall, and the pair of them came in and heaved her up.

She's been taught how to get up, but you have to be near something to get up, and if you try often enough you get tired, you just don't have the strength to do it. Anyway, we've managed so far, and she's got a call button.

If I were to advise carers, I suppose it's a question of your relationship before you start out. We were very good friends, which I can't say we are now! She's fed up to the back teeth with me. There's nothing I can do about it. She's stuck with me, and I'm stuck here, that's it, get on with it. There's no point in moaning about it, you just pick up your bootlaces and get on. Keep your sense of humour, most important. We still laugh at the same things.

I suppose, try and get breaks though it's all very well saying that, but it doesn't work out that way. If her friend comes down, she'll come on a Saturday or a Sunday and then go back the following week. I feel I've got to be here when she comes and when she goes, so I've only got those days in between, which is not much time to really get away.

Each of you needs a break from each other. I don't work physically hard, because we have carers coming in, morning and evening, so that's not the problem. It's just the general feeling of having to make all the decisions. I know I don't - she hasn't lost her brainpower - but you do feel a bit alone sometimes; but that's it.

The most important thing I suppose is just to be here. When she falls, or drops something. So there's always somebody here. I tell her she's lucky to have me! In her heart she knows, I hope, but I've been here virtually since she had her stroke, which was in 2012. That's over four years.

I've never been much for gadding around, neither my late husband nor myself. We had lovely holidays in our camper van, and we used to go off frequently, all over Britain and the Continent. But we never went shopping or anything, just for the sake of going out; we've never done that. Even my GP says, why don't you join a carers' group, but I'm not a socialising person; that doesn't worry me. I'm very self-sufficient. I can amuse myself; I don't need to see anyone for days; it doesn't bother me. Because I can do things I want to do. So that side of it doesn't worry me. I don't hanker to go out anywhere. I know these groups are very helpful to some people, but not for me.

I potter, even on my own at home. I read. I do my crosswords, my code words. I like my garden – of course I've taken over this garden. I have some help now, someone who comes in every couple of weeks, or during the growing season. Of course I had friends and I've had to leave them all behind. They're all 'old', or they're not quite fit to travel too often to see us.

I've always said if your back's to the wall you're on your own. That's very sad, but it's perfectly true. And I've told my daughter right from childhood, don't rely on other people. You've got to be yourself. Obviously you ask for help if you really need to, but when crunch-time comes you're on your own. It's not fair to rely on others to make decisions for you. I know going to these groups is very helpful to lots of people, but not for me. I have got very good friends; we're all nurses and we support each other when necessary.

WILL STAMMERS

Will Stammers had a high-flying job in the defence industry moving explosives around the world. It required expertise and knowledge to follow complex international safety protocols.

Since Will's stroke his son, according to Will's mum, says his Dad 'forgets a lot of things'. Unlike so many stroke survivors, Will is physically very active. He rides his bike regularly, but does admit to getting very tired. As a committee member and trustee of Stroke Club, UK, Will is adamant just how stroke survivors should be treated by the wider community. Here is Will's story:

I was active; I used to enjoy going out on my bike. I didn't do running or anything like that, but I used to enjoy being active. I used to go to the gym when I was working, because the gym was a few doors down from where I used to work: Logistics; complicated logistics; movement of weapons; explosives from A to B. So, all the legislation around that is very complicated, and engulfing, in what you can and can't do. There are some parts, official secrets, I can't tell you exactly what I used to do, but basically movement of defence material from A to B, around the world - from the States to Australia, from the UK to Australia, and say, UK businesses to Europe.

I know exactly why I had my stroke. It was in 2011, I was thirty-eight – I'm now forty-two. It was due to Antiphospolipid Syndrome (APS), or Hughes Syndrome, which is an auto-immune condition that makes your blood sticky and clot easily. Also I had the high blood pressure associated with that, so we believe that there was a clot lying around in my body somewhere that moved up to my brain.

Six months before I now believe I had a TIA: purely because they could see it on my MRI scan. Around October I had severe dizziness, throwing up one day: I couldn't stand up properly without falling over. But the GP didn't realise that. He gave me anti-dizziness pills; said 'you'll be fine', and sent me away again. I don't believe he linked that I had the clotting thing, with the dizziness, or expected it to be a TIA.

The actual stroke, with hindsight, we believe happened during the night, purely because we can't pin down when the stroke actually happened to me. A February morning, about an inch of snow on the ground, I got up for work, same as I did every other day, on a Friday morning, cleared the snow off the drive, cleared the cars, the snow and drove to work.

And then when I got to work people said to me, 'your face is a bit puffy, are you all right?' I said 'I feel fine', which I did, I felt fine. 'Your speech sounds a bit slurred.' I said, 'does it, I feel fine'. They said 'are you sure you're all right?' I said, 'yes, fine'. They happened to know about my APS. They said, 'you're really not right, let's get you down to the doctors'. So I went down to the local doctors in Wallingford where I was working, and the doctor said, 'no, you're really not right; I think you've had a stroke'. Okay, so from there the doctor called an ambulance and I went straight to the JR (John Radcliffe Hospital) in Oxford.

They did an initial assessment; the usual tests; the holding hands out in front of you to see if you are deficient down one side, that sort of thing. Gripping things, you know, 'can you grip my two fingers?' All the usual tests, which I believe are normal for someone they think has had a stroke: touch your nose; follow the pen with your eye.

I was in hospital for seven days, mainly because I was actually living in Northampton at the time, even though I was in an Oxfordshire hospital, because I was working in Oxfordshire. (I used to commute about sixty miles a day, there and back - sixty miles each way.)

I was initially very slurry at hospital, the first week afterwards, but I could speak. It took me a long while to get words out, and make up a proper sentence but I could do it after a while. Part of my therapy they gave me a picture board of a lot of different pictures, and say, what's that, what's that? Okay, now remember what's on that picture board. So they were quite intensive in that respect, maybe because they realised I was young and my brain was quite malleable at that time; so it could be formed into a shape there and then, at the early stages, which is most important to make it more effective for my recovery.

I got released after a week from the JR. They were initially worried about my swallowing, because they don't want you to swallow and choke, and have pneumonia or something. That was their initial concern, me swallowing properly, before I could be let out on my own. But Northamptonshire actually has a very good community stroke team that comes round to your house every day, which I believe is quite a rare thing. I don't know the stats and stuff.

So I was released under their care, and they would come and see me everyday to do various things: physio, speech and language therapy, to try and get me up to speed as quickly as possible, which I think helped tremendously. I think that's a plan they should try to do, try to convince the health authorities that it's a good idea, to get people home in the home environment, where they feel comfortable, to do things they would do normally every day. Things like, if you've got a gammy hand, you try to spread butter on your toast. How do you do that? Spread jam on a bit of toast, you can't do it, when you've only got one hand. Put your socks on with one hand; tie your shoelaces with one hand.

I still had the use of my left hand, even though it was left side affected, but only very basically. If they got me to turn my hand over, it would often fall back down: the basic grasp function to drink a cup of tea. My hand is still weak, and I notice it if I'm carrying two cups of tea, I'll spill more.

I was married, two children, newborn, six months old. I think Susan managed okay. Living not far from her relatives we had quite a strong family network immediately in the vicinity. So they were happy to help quite a lot. Did the kids notice? They were probably a little bit too young to fully appreciate what was going on. They knew that daddy hadn't been very well, was in hospital, and of course they came to see me in hospital, but I don't think they really appreciated what happened. Probably to their benefit I think.

Initially I was off work for about three months. Then from that they allowed me to do a phased return; like a day a week, then maybe two days a week, three days a week, etc. It was very difficult because at that time I couldn't drive, because I didn't feel confident enough to drive, so someone had to take me to work. So my mum and dad took me to work; they'd spend the day in Wallingford, walk round the village, the town, then come and pick me up at the end of the day, and take me home.

After that it's up to you to decide if you can drive. It transpired after a few months I went to the doctor and said, 'do you think I'm safe to drive?' And they said, 'can you see?' Vision tests. And said 'I can't see any problem why you shouldn't drive'.

I was extremely tired. Everything being thrown at you at what you believe is two hundred miles an hour and you've got to process it. The whole decision-making process is slower than it used to be. I can appreciate now that it's slower than it used to be. It's taking on information, particularly when you're driving, because you've got 360 degrees to concentrate on, trying to concentrate on that all at the same time, and make sensible informed decisions. Like, are you going to stop, are you going to go? All those things make a really heavy load on the brain.

Work ended for me; work was very legislation-based, what you can and can't do moving sensitive explosive material around. You've got to remember that, and of course when you've had a stroke and you've got to take it all on board again, trying to make those connections. In logistics, if you're trying to plan moving things from A to B, if something goes wrong half-way down A, how is that going to affect things further on? The load on your brain trying to understand the knock on effects, I could only do it to a certain extent. Work recognised that and took me to the office one day and said, 'look, it's not working is it? So I think you should go'.

It was painful. It hurt very much not being able to work. There we go. It happens. It is very much a stroke club mantra, 'shit happens'. It was a very small company, only about a half a dozen people in the office, so trying to find a niche for someone with limited skills, if you want to call it that, would have been very difficult. I got a bit of severance pay after advice from a solicitor.

My short-term memory has disappeared, that sort of thing. Things like your mental chatter in your brain - all these things going on in your mind all the time- it was like the phone is switched off. Where has all the chatter gone? Really quiet. So in a way quite eerie is the silence that you can feel. Where ideas came into your head all the time, it's just switched off. It wasn't disconcerting because I didn't really notice it. But having read the book 'My Stroke of Insight' by Jill Bolte Taylor, PhD, I said, yes, I agree with that. That's why I can't make similes and parallels.

I think I was a bright person, intelligent. If I seem like it now that veil is working! A little bit behind a persona, because having the two kids you try to juggle so many things that you try and remember everything, even like walking out the door in the morning: have you got the kids' lunch, got the kids' water bottles; got their jackets, got their hats, have you put sun cream on them? All these things you've got to try and think about before you leave the house. Only when you're driving to school you think, 'oh, forgotten that'! Or, 'have I remembered to pay a bill, empty the bins, put the washing out?' Can be stressful.

I think one of my primary feelings now is, I often feel useless, and my confidence has been degraded by my often failings: like forgetting things. It chips away at your confidence, but I haven't dwelled on what I miss because there's lots about it I can't change. One circle of thought, why dwell on the things you can't have, or you're not going to have. What's the point? What are you going to gain from that? Probably, before, when I was working full time, before I had my stroke, I guess the hunter-gatherer mentality, I was working, supporting the family, and I was lucky enough to be in a position where I could support the family. My wife didn't have to go out to work, even though she was fully capable of working. In that interim period she had to find employment; that was the role reversal.

I don't mind that she has gone out to work now – she is Depot Manager for the John Lewis home delivery service in West London. It's her career. She can do what she wants. If that's what she wants to do, fair play. I wish I could do it. Do I put on the big man act: I should be earning the money; I should be doing things around the house, or do I just let her do it? A side of me has resigned myself; I can't do it as well as I used to, so she can do it if she's happy enough to do it. We're very lucky to know as well that what I used to earn and what she earns now, we can both support the family with just one person earning; we both fully realise we're very lucky to do that.

I do volunteering at the school for young eight year olds, which for me if very good for learning. Like, they're learning about adverbs, onomatopoeic words: young children they're such sponges. I don't remember learning at school what a subordinate clause was. So those things I've re-learned have been really good. Then when you try to tell it to other people it concretes your learning and understanding of it. So for me that has been a really valuable aspect, learning from fresh.

Stroke Club Didcot, we're a bunch of sixty or seventy members, meetings normally consist of about two dozen; people have had strokes at various times of their lives. Some of them have only had strokes, say, about a year ago. There's one guy who comes in who's younger than me - I think he's mid-twenties - he had a stroke when he was four. So of course he doesn't really know anything different.

We sit in a very sociable atmosphere, i.e the pub, whether you drink or whatever, that's your choice. A lot of people think, 'shit happens', shall I drink or shan't I? Can this get any worse? No, let's have a beer then. So there is that kind of line of thought with some people, but some people will have coffee, like me, I normally have a soda lime. I normally drink soft drinks; I'm driving as well. And I will get very tired if I have a couple of beers as well. Then it's game over!

If I'm here on my own, the kids are at school, I'll either go on my bike for a couple of hours, do twenty miles on my bike; luckily enough I didn't have problems with my balance. Or, if I'm feeling particularly shattered one day, for whatever reason, then I'll just go and have a kip.

My wife is not my carer; she's my ally. I don't think of her as my carer because I can do pretty much everything I used to. Only cognitive things, if things build up, they take a while to process and when they do process lights come on everywhere: I should have said that, should have said this. I wasn't able to read at first then I could. Some words are slower to understand, their full meaning, but I could read. I nap very well and generally sleep well. Sometimes I wake up with various aches and pains, probably from the medication I'm on, like cramps and things like that.

The first year after my stroke travel insurance was about four hundred quid a year. Now going away this year it's gone down to about two hundred pounds. As time goes on it's decreasing. But it probably isn't helped that I had a fit as well. I had a fit about eighteen months after my stroke. I believe a third of stroke survivors have a fit within eighteen months/two years of having a stroke.

I was in the shower and I felt fine, ready to go out for the day. Everyone was downstairs, my wife, my outlaws, the kids. My wife said she heard the shower door open and close and after that all she heard was a juddering noise. I didn't know anything about it; I was out of it. What it was, I was hanging on to the enamel sink and fitting.

My wife came upstairs to see what was happening. She hadn't a clue what was going on; she wasn't aware a fit was possible. I fell forward, struck my chest on the taps – I've got a scar here on my chest – and started to keel over. She was holding me, trying to stop me smashing my head. My whole body was tensing up, wasn't even breathing. She got me down on the floor and screamed for her mum and dad to help her. I was starting to go blue, but from there I started to come round a bit and started to breathe again. For her that was probably the most frightening thing for her throughout all of this.

I have a very full life. Two children growing up fast, too fast, all parents say that. My elder daughter wants to be a brain surgeon.

Whether that's been affected by my experience, probably not. We have explained to her what a stroke is, what it does. Now being eight she can understand it a bit more now.

I think I personally have quite a positive outlook on life, but whether that's my age or whatever, I don't know. I think I'm quite naturally like that, which I think has been a big help in the way I've got through this. Being a positive person helps no end. One of the few things I remember in hospital they said, 'what goals have you got in the future?' One of the things I said was that I wanted to pick up my boy - which I realised at the time was a realistic goal. It wasn't pie in the sky, like to be an astronaut. I didn't want anything more than that: I just wanted to pick up my boy. Now I just pick him up.

Susan has been a rock. She understands everything I have been through and the problems of having a stroke. We often have a laugh that as my memory has been affected, whenever we visit places that I have been before it is a brand new experience every time!

So did I get off lightly with my stroke? Yes. Through the stroke club I met a lot of people who didn't get off so lightly. People in wheelchairs, people limping, people who can't talk properly. Does it boost my morale seeing those people? Not really, no. I want to see those people get better. I want to try and help them improve. I don't long for a cure, why should I? Because I know there isn't one. A key thing for me is to keep fit, keep on top of any ailments; look after your body. You've only got one, live in it.

Stroke club is very positive in terms of people who have come off a lot worse than you; you want to help them progress. That is very satisfying; not make people better but make their lives better. To anyone who has just had a stroke, I'd say, 'I've been there. Is it hard? Yes. Will it be hard? Yes. Will you get over it? Yes. Can you do it? Yes'.

It's a journey. All the shit you go through; the pain it causes everyone around you. I fully believe that anyone who hasn't had a stroke, and aren't close to us family-wise have absolutely no idea what's involved. Friends and stuff can sympathise, but do they empathise? I certainly find that my level of empathy for other people has skyrocketed. It has for both of us. When you see people with difficulties trying to do things, you're level of empathy is phenomenal. The stroke club is more about empathy than sympathy, because it is run by stroke survivors.

That's one thing we're trying to conquer. The acute stroke ward in the JR; at the moment they won't let you go on the ward because they've got contractual things; sensitivity because of records flying around. But I'm currently in dialogue with them, trying to get on the ward as a volunteer, so I can sit beside someone's bed and say, 'hi, I've been there; I've got the t-shirt'.

*www.strokeclubuk.org

HEATHER LAWRENCE

Heather was a Deputy Head who spent a good part of her career in private education. Since her stroke, Heather has been looked after by her husband David, who is now her registered carer.

Reverend Canon David Lawrence was a Church of England vicar at the time of Heather's stroke. I feel his career definitely prepared him for his role as carer. He is secretary and an active committee member of the local Stroke Club.

Every week they kindly give me a lift into Stroke club. They are a devoted couple and the journey is always full of light-hearted conversation. Here is Heather's story:

I was the same person as I am now with physical disabilities. I still am a wife, a mother and a grandmother.

My mother wanted me to be a secretary; my father said I should be an engineer. So I went and studied zoology and chemistry at university. Got married while I was still at university, and we had our first daughter. I had no idea what to do for a job or career. I got a job lecturing in what is now a university but was then a technical college and went on from there: a series of teaching posts, in prisons, schools. Then I got a job in a private school and stayed in the private sector, which I enjoyed very much, getting paid a lot less, surprisingly. I did that for thirty-one years.

Latterly I had been getting a little irate with the post I had; I was Head of Science at a girls' school: and I wasn't too keen on the headmistress - most of that probably my fault. But she was chatting up the head of Cheltenham College and said she had someone who she thought suitable for this live-in job. So I went for an interview there on a Sunday morning.

All the then head wanted to know was my attitude towards sex and drugs. I thought, yes, that's an interesting interview! But I went into the garden with his wife, and I thought anyone who has such an amazingly wonderful wife can't be all bad. And I'd heard he was an incredibly eloquent speaker publicly, and his vision was amazing so I did accept the job. I noticed they didn't have suitable drainpipes for boys to get into the girls' house so I thought, yes, I can do this job.

The first term I don't think I slept; just worrying the whole time what was going to happen. I was House Mistress in charge of a brand new boarding house for girls seventeen to twenty-one - because the Asian girls were always a bit older. It was all alarmed and I knew they were safe, but I didn't sleep for a whole term, I eventually calmed down.

It worked and I enjoyed it. David had his vicarage and we had this thing where we saw each other at least once a day, so it might have been breakfast, it might have been lunch, it might have been supper. He'd occasionally climb over the wall and spend the night with me. And I would have a day off a week, and night off, because you didn't just run a house, I taught Biology and a little Chemistry as well, and that worked okay.

Eventually I ran four houses, had four housemistresses, and after five years they wanted to make me what they called Senior Mistress. By this time I was on my third headmaster and I thought, no, I'm nobody's mistress unless I choose to be. So I decided to be Senior Teacher, which I suppose is equivalent to Deputy Head Pastoral in the State school. I moved out of the House and when we moved to the Forest of Dean – when David took a Parish out there - I'd drive thirty-four miles each way to work. I enjoyed what I did, responsible for new teachers, all new pupils and all child protection issues.

I was there when we introduced the first girl. Obviously it was difficult because girls' prep schools kept their girls until they were eleven, and they then went on to a girls' school. Whereas the boys' prep schools kept them until thirteen, so we had our first young girl at thirteen. She became the very first head girl of the school: the senior pupil. In my career I taught all girls; all boys; co-ed, so I felt I had a handle at what was going on.

I retired at the end of the academic year, when I was sixty. I made an effort to stay reasonably healthy. Our vicarage was on the top of a hill of a little town, and I would walk down to the town every day, and do shopping, and come back with my back loaded with my two bags of shopping. One Saturday I was feeling particularly tired coming back from a shopping expedition. And on the Sunday I distinctly remember, church in the morning, lunch, and I'd promised a lady to take her swimming.

I began to feel a little bit not quite right, but I was meant to be the one caring for her – she had a bad back – so I was trying to ring someone else up to see if they would take her swimming. I just could not hold the telephone directory. I dropped it and ran to the lavatory and knew things were not quite right. Then David came in and took one look at me and dialled 999: 'my wife's had a stroke'.

I don't think I lost consciousness. They tried to put me in a chair to take me to the ambulance. My face had gone and I'd lost all the strength in my left hand - although I could still talk. (David says it will freeze over in hell before I stop talking! He probably means it as well!)

They keep asking you the same questions: like, who is the Prime Minister? Do you care who the Prime Minister is! Do you have a headache, do you have this; do you have that? I couldn't move; I was actually quite immobile. It was explained later that I had atrial fibrilation. You have four main chambers: your left and right atrium, your left and right ventricles. If the atrium beats out of rhythm you have an automatic pacemaker that keeps you going, and it was not beating correctly. It caused the blood to swirl and as it did that it caused a clot and the clot then got shot into my brain, lodged in one of the cranial arteries. It then deprives parts of the brain of oxygen and then it dies.

Then, with all the tissue damage, your brain starts to swell and as it pushes on the cerebellum, which is the base of the brain and essential for automatic functions: heart beat, breathing. I was getting to the stage of no heartbeat, no breathing, and you don't go on much longer. David was told basically she's going to die, but he said 'there must be something you can do'.

I had a cerebral accident. With a physiology degree I'm quite comfortable with the language. They told him that a craniotomy can take some of the skull away to relieve the pressure, but I was too old. The chances of survival aren't great and the chance of even more damage is great. David said 'if there's a chance we ought to take the chance. She's very fit; she's very determined; she's never smoked'. He didn't lie and say I'd never drunk. I think probably I'd drunk too much. I think that was probably the issue: I'd drunk too much. I'd had a stressful job, which I loved, and I did three hundred miles a week just getting to and from school. I think those things were significant.

They took me down to Frenchay Hospital, Bristol: the team there agreed to have a go at it. Apparently it was a long night for David. They operated most of the night; took away probably a third, a fair chunk, of my cranium and I've still got all the scars under the amazing amount of hair I still have. I was sixty-one. I wasn't frightened. Fear's a funny thing. I'm always fearful when I go under anaesthetic. *(Heather weeps)* It's just that David would not give me the last rites. I told him to do that. He said you don't have to do that.

They still kept asking who the Prime Minister was. I still didn't really care, and now I care even less! I wore a medical helmet for a year; you know like a bicycle helmet; actually more like a boxer's helmet. I had no cranium so I wasn't allowed to move until they made it exactly the right size for my head or it's not going to work. I wasn't allowed out of bed, but eventually after ages I got the helmet, and was allowed into a wheelchair and go to the loo. (I had to learn to pee again after a catheter!)

I had the helmet for a year and eventually got my plate. January 2011 was the stroke; February 2012 was when I had the titanium plate put in. We went to stay with our younger daughter in

Swindon, to be closer to Bristol for stitches and staples to be taken out.

In the October in the year of the stroke I had quite a serious seizure. We had two grandchildren here so it must have been half term. It started in a very strange way. I don't remember a lot of that. Again David got the ambulance because he said this is not right; I don't know if it's another stroke. They couldn't stop it. I woke up with all the patches on me; shocking me, and I had lots of injections. They took me off to Dorchester. That was not a very good experience; I didn't enjoy that at all.

The explanation for that is, if you have fits or seizures straight after a stroke it's the effect of the initial brain damage. You recover from that and don't tend to have them again. If you have a late onset seizure, which is what mine was, it's the indication of deeper brain damage. My physiotherapist here said we call what you experienced *Alice in Wonderland Syndrome*. Lewis Caroll had this disorder where he saw things growing. I saw people shrinking in front of my eyes; and auditory hallucinations, which again is due to brain damage. Most often with this syndrome, people grow, but with me they shrank, which is rare.

It was a little distressing for a while. When we came home I could hear the car radio and it wasn't on. And I could hear the television and it wasn't on. That went on for a while and then it stopped. I must admit I needed David a lot then, just for a touch of reality. I'm quite sensitive to certain things. That didn't last too long. I'm on epileptic drugs to stop that kind of thing.

We had to have adaptations for creature comfort, so I could climb the stairs to bed. I could move around, and I couldn't really go without my helmet because your brain is exposed and very vulnerable. I had flesh on it obviously; they pull your scalp back over. I couldn't get out of bed without a helmet on.

Someone would collect me and take me to church on Sunday because I couldn't find the edge of things easily. Part of that was to do with sight problems anyway, but I wasn't good at that. It was limited movement and I had all that physiotherapy game: the local Forest of Dean hospital had a physio department and I would go there fortnightly, weekly or whatever.

Physically I was a bit limited, but before I left hospital I was walking. I used the wheelchair, which was fine, but I was irritated with that and then the physio said let's try the stick. David says my spatial awareness was never any good and I really couldn't manage the stick and two legs. So we just said – and the children remember - we used to say 'left right, left right' and I could do it. My movements are not too bad. Obviously I couldn't walk anywhere, couldn't go anywhere on my own.

So physically I was a bit limited. I had a very good stroke nurse; she was lovely: and a totally useless occupational therapist. One shouldn't knock the NHS - they have the most horrendous workloads. She came out with her notepad – we were just having lunch at the time – could I cook lunch? At that stage I could not use my left hand at all, so I couldn't hold a knife. I'm still banned from knives. I can cut but I don't do much - although I haven't to date cut myself - but then, he keeps sharpening the knives!

My eldest daughter who is a children's occupational therapist, said 'mum there are all these aids for cutting. They're not available on the NHS but you can buy them'. So there were plenty of things we could do to solve things and I had a fat knife and fork I could use.

The stroke was what it was, which is mostly my attitude to life: it is what it is. My daughter in law said, 'aren't you angry that it happened?' And I said, 'why?' In fact I was put in my place well and truly, by the lady whose husband had died in the January of that year from his stroke. They would say to her, 'Aren't you angry that Heather has survived, and your husband didn't?' She said, 'No. Of course I didn't want Chris to die. I didn't want Heather to die either.' And I'm thinking, 'wow, that's really where it's at'.

I wouldn't want anyone but David as my carer. I'm a pretty tetchy person. I wouldn't want anyone else to come in and bath me, wash me. I can get in the bath, but I can't get out. I trust him implicitly. He's been there for the birth of three children; there's not much he doesn't know about me.

I have an expectation that David would have looked after me no matter what, and insisted that he was registered officially as my carer. Not that he needed the money, but we then get the carer's support. It's jumping through hoops to get what is yours, which is what my first stroke nurse did for us. We would not claim disability because we said we don't need it. He said 'that's true now but you don't know what's going to happen; you don't know how this is going to progress'. He was a savvy man.

I feel I'd like David to be freer. Not being totally tied by everything he says he has to do. Which is why I insisted that we had a cleaner come in again. Obviously we had cleaners when I worked because I couldn't do working and cleaning because I was never there.

He does everything. He gets me up. He walks the dog. Everything revolves around where you can go and what you can do. I can imagine how carers could feel resentful. David was ill a little while back – he was off work for six months; he'd been in hospital - he says only two weeks, I think a bit longer than that -

and he was very difficult to look after. He's been ill twice in his life and I remember on both those occasions being quite resentful about him being ill. So I could see he could be resentful having to look after me, although in fairness he never shows that. But I can understand it.

My raison d'etre is to say there's always hope. No matter what, you mustn't lose hope. And enjoy who you are and what you have. You may feel like it's not very much. My mother in law said 'oh it can't get any worse'. And I thought, 'don't be stupid it can always get worse'. So I think, hang on to the good bits. And there are good bits. I have only to think of, say, Molly (name changed) at Stroke Club who is trapped in her soundless world. Her brain works; she understands what you say to her. She lives on her own and is very lonely. Yet she has joy in seeing people, and she remembers people. The cognition is there, and she knows what she's doing. It's just the words will not come, and they are never going to come.

But I'm a great believer in neuroplasticity, that the brain will transfer one function to another. Even if you are very old it does work. And it's all right to be afraid that you'll have more strokes because you are probably likely to. All the more reason to enjoy what you've got, because you do not know what's around the corner. Psalms said, this is the day the Lord has made. Let us rejoice in it gladly - because tomorrow you could be screwed (I added that bit myself!). You just don't know.

Your relationships with other people, how other people view you. I don't have an issue with that. In fact, having said that, I obviously do, because people do view me differently. I was explaining to someone on Sunday that what people do now is knock on the door and say 'here's a book, you might like to read it'. As opposed to saying 'would you like to come out and play'? I don't get out to play any more. I miss all that. I miss the camaraderie of being with other people. But then David and I planned a retirement pre the stroke. We knew what we were doing, moving away from all the people we knew to be together and do things. But then I can't because of my physical limitations and because of the dogs we can't do a lot of things.

I want to visit Hardy's house; just had a whole session reading Hardy again. We can't go because you can't take dogs. We can walk in the woods but I can't walk very far. People who are brave enough to visit me: my old secretary comes down once a year and because my gob is as ever was they feel I haven't changed in what I say and what I do.

And I still go to my book club. We're a group of ladies of a certain age. There's only one unmarried and she says I haven't missed as much as I think I might have missed. They were ones who visited me in hospital, took me out straight afterwards when I really was quite limited. David trusted them to take me out. It's good to go and talk to them and not be treated differently. They'll help me go to the loo; they are thoughtful. One had polio as a child and has a leg iron.

Stroke Club gives an element of continuity, and I'm a great believer in continuity. I trust people who remain the same. If people are awful, but are consistently awful, I have respect for people who have consistency. I've a lot of respect for some of the helpers there. Some of them have been quite ill themselves, and are still quite ill. I'm just amazed they give so willingly of their time to do what they do.

And I miss one of the ladies who used to be there, far more physically disabled than I am, but had emotional intelligence and was someone I could actually share thoughts with. But now there's no one to talk to now.

There are some regrets. I can't do things I planned to do, but we might do them if we move to Bristol. We have to move somewhere bigger to do some of the things I want to do. I could use the Open University, but I like people, I want to be with people.

I'm grateful for retaining my brain, and to the old guy for looking after me. And caring.

My brother looks after his wife, and he says he doesn't know how David does what he does. David looks after me and still has an emotional attachment to me. My brother says he's quite capable of looking after his wife physically, but the emotional attachment he says he finds hard. So I'm grateful – for having it all really. I can't run a marathon, but then I never wanted to run a marathon: never ever.

David says:

Stroke club gives stroke survivors an outlet where they don't have to pretend to be well and a hundred percent able-bodied. Not everyone knows what it's like to have a stroke and the devastation of that, how that changes you. I think Stroke club is a safe place where you can be who you are without let or hindrance.

Routinely I suppose I help Heather with getting dressed; with all the hygiene stuff, including showering; cooking. I do the garden. We used to do that as a team but it now more or less all falls to me. I do cop out and get other people in to do bits for us from time to time. So I don't do as many DIY things as I used to, simply because I don't have the time.

I don't feel tied, not really. I say not really because initially it was such a shock and I didn't quite know what Heather would be able to do coming out of the stroke, recovering. And because she had a craniectomy for a year she had a kind of crash helmet and also didn't have the use of her left hand and arm very much. So there was an exploration as to how much movement and things she would get back in that, and so on. So it was a question of gently, gently.

I suppose in that period I felt tied, but also wanted to be tied, because I didn't want to let other people in, in case they triggered something that would go wrong. So at the end of a year when Heather had the cranioplasty I felt a lot more relaxed, because we had moved down here to Lyme. I didn't have any ties to the Parish any longer and I could just spend all my time looking after her.

With a Parish you have to be on duty all the time. I had a staff team of four Readers, as well as seven others to organise, seeing them off to do bits. Other times they would be self-motivated enough to get on and do it themselves. But it was just keeping everything together, because we were a very busy Parish. We had about forty weddings a year. We had a wedding venue in the parish and three pretty churches and people wanted to get married in them. So we would find ways of allowing that to happen, which meant we made commitments to doing prep and getting really involved.

As Heather's carer I do have time to myself. On Friday nights, I decided I wanted to do something different, so I now sing with the Lyme Regis shanty singers *Harbour Voices*. Not every Friday night, but this weekend we're singing at Trill, a venue up the road.

Sunday 30 January 2011, the day of the stroke, I'd just finished Evensong, and as I was coming out of the church, I wondered whether to go home or see one of our treasurers whose husband had died three weeks earlier, and who I hadn't seen that morning. I thought, 'I'm tired I'm going home to see Heather'. Luckily, because I arrived home about 5pm and she'd actually had the stroke about ten minutes earlier.

I walked in just after she'd had it. We were coming here to Lyme for a few days off and the bags were packed in the hall. The light was on in the study, books on the floor, which I couldn't understand. I called her, but no answer. The light was on in the kitchen, but she wasn't there. Then I heard a noise from the toilet round the corner and she was there, looking confused and her mouth had gone. I immediately knew what she had.

She'd had a bit of an accident; she'd had the stroke and was still conscious, so I helped get her cleaned up and immediately called 999.

I was shocked, but I went into the mode of, I know what this is, this is the mode I've got to be in. I had seen it previously when my mother had had a stroke when I was in visiting her in hospital.

Heather instantly got carted off to Gloucester Royal. I ran round, got together a small bag, some water, and followed her in. By the time I got there she had already been scanned, a CT scan, and they found it was a stroke. There was a blood clot that had gone up to her brain, and they could tell you where it was at the top. She still had this amazing headache, and I sat with her a bit. Then they said, 'we're going to give this injection to break up the clot'. But the consultant decided against it because the x-ray showed a little bit of bleeding around the clot. It would be dangerous to give the anti-coagulant because that could cause something massive. So they gave pain relief, and said 'let's see how this goes on'.

I got kicked out; I couldn't stay the night because she went into the Medical Admissions ward. I was extremely anxious because with my job as a vicar I had lots of experience with patients who died of a stroke. I'd also worked in a path lab. So the next day when I saw her I was shocked because she was going more into a comatose sort of state. She said she had this pounding headache, and had managed to break a glass. In letting her go to the toilet on her own, it had fallen off as she stumbled through the door.

I was unhappy with the ward she was in; unhappy with the state she was getting in. I think visiting time was 2.30 until about 4pm, and 5.30 to 7.30, something like that, so it was a split shift. I sat with her, talked a bit, she talked a bit, but was getting a bit slurry in her speech and tired. Her eyes kept going and she'd doze off and come back again.

That was the first bit and the second bit, she was obviously very unwell and was going deeper into this kind of coma thing. So I went and had a go at the consultant and said, 'I don't like this at all', and she said, 'oh well, we'll just wait and see'. And I said, 'it's not good enough really. You know and I know she's dying, and this can only go one way. Are we going to sit here and watch her die? I'm not happy, and that's how it is. Is there nothing else that can be done at this stage?'

She said, 'well there is an operation they can do, but I think she's probably too old for that', and we went through the thing about her age and how fit she had been, and she was just retired. She was sixty-one, which was just over the top limit, and then the consultant said, 'what I'll do, I'll send her CT scans down to Bristol and they can make a decision. It's down to them. It's not down to me; I can agree to send it'.

So that was about 4 o'clock I suppose. We sat there and sat there and Heather was getting worse and I had to nudge her a bit; saying 'Oi, you all right mate, how you doing?' all that sort of stuff. 'Don't go to sleep on me. I'm not visiting you here for nothing. I expect you to talk to me. Speak to me woman.' And she'd say…'sorrrrry' or whatever. By 8 o'clock nothing had happened, and I went back and the consultant said, 'ah, well, this is what has happened. I'm about to go off duty'. This was the Monday night now, and eventually she went off at about 10 o'clock but she again phoned Bristol and said 'the guys are in the theatre. I've told my registrar and she will come back to you as soon as they contact us'.

Around 11 o'clock, after the consultant had gone off, the registrar came back and said they would take Heather down to Bristol, but were waiting for transport. By this time my anxiety was stratospheric I suppose. I could just see her not making it, because she was beginning to go into this comatose state. Her breathing was getting more erratic. Then suddenly this nurse who I'd had a fight with, came in and said 'oh I've got to give her this', and had a shunt, you know, one of those butterfly things they shove into your arm, and started trying to squeeze this stuff in. Then blokes turned up with a trolley, and half of it went in and half didn't.

They transferred her to the trolley, and wheeled her out fast and went off, blue-lighted, down to Bristol. I jumped in the car and stopped at the petrol station in what, in fact, was my first parish where I was a curate. I bought myself one of those energy drink things; a Redbull - I thought I'd probably need to stay awake tonight – and a sandwich.

My daughter had been with us at the Gloucester Royal hospital; she'd gone about 10 o'clock. Our other daughter who was nine months pregnant hadn't come to the hospital; she couldn't face it. And my son was in South Africa. I phoned him and I said 'I think mum's dying, so prepare yourself for bad news'. I got to Frenchay hospital. She arrived and I spoke to the registrar and the anaesthetist, and he had noticed Heather wasn't breathing properly. I wanted to shake her and say 'breathe will you, breathe'!

My daughter had arrived by this time – she came straight back. It was then about half past one, and Heather went to theatre then. There were two people in front of her, but they realised she was so bad they put her in first. And actually it was quite amazing because this guy with a great long Indian name, who called himself Sunni, he took me to one side and I just felt almost completely at peace. All my anxiety just kind of poured out of me, because he obviously knew exactly what he was doing and gave me absolute confidence. I knew she was in the right place; and I couldn't do more. It was brilliant.

I suppose I was just incredibly grateful for the whole thing, because it was so, so good. I can't praise them enough. And Heather came back onto the ward about half past eight, and she was then high-dependency, connected to a machine that went beep because her heart had done a funny flutter. Later in the morning it was slowed down because it was beating too fast. Gave her some *Digoxin* and shut the whole thing down. But apart from that the next week went by very quickly. They got her up and out of bed by the end of that week, which was amazing.

But it was also weird. By then my son had arrived from South Africa and I had him to look after as well; which was a good distraction, bless him. People in South Africa were praying for her and the Bishop had come to see her. And I knew - being a Canon and things - all the people in the Cathedral chapter were praying for her. You know what I mean, I felt surrounded with support and the rest of my team back in the parish were actually looking after it really well. And the hard bit was actually just keeping up with all her buddies and friends, when I came back from visiting the hospital because there would be a hundred emails.

So I said, 'look, you guys, can you have one person who can send it on to everyone?' So I nominated two or three people, so I didn't spend all the rest of the night doing things. So that was easy; I was just looking after myself really. And we didn't have dogs then so it was really very easy.

My sense of the extent of my need to care happened even at Bristol. By day three the registrar said 'I need to talk to you', and took us into the office. He said 'it's hard for you because you've been sitting at home, but I need to show you the CT scan'. So he showed us the scan and there's a track through the brain obviously in layers. You could see this massive area; she'd effectively lost the frontal right lobe, and he said 'she's going to be pretty disabled; we don't know yet how much. It's about how much care she'll need'. He was trying to gently tell me that she would be a vegetable.

I felt 'you're wrong mate', because she was already communicating quite lucidly and getting p'eed off with people. And compared to some of the people I had already known who had strokes who couldn't speak or couldn't swallow – in two days her swallow had come back; it wasn't strong but it was back. So by about day three or four she began to have mushed-up food; and soups and that kind of thing. So all the signs were good, and by the end of the week he said to me 'I can't believe how well she's done in a week. She's very strong in her legs, and I'm sure she'll walk soon.'

The next thing was she got transferred back to Gloucester, and the first three weeks there were a nightmare because she couldn't do anything. She had to stay in bed because she didn't have the safety helmet. So it was like three weeks in limbo, but then they put all the physios onto her and within a week she was walking up and down the corridor on her own. Her speech had come back completely. Her hand wasn't back, but we were working on her hand and trying to get her to wriggle her fingers and things. Her bladder was good. Her bowels were working okay. All the normal functions were normal.

When it first happened I remember being quite angry, and also kind of praying saying 'hey boss, what are you doing. I can't go through this now. You can't take her away in my last year when I've got all these other things; I just won't be able to cope. I'll have to chuck it up. I won't be able to look after six churches and a big parish.' And I felt supported by God, so I think my faith helped me in all of that.

I think the next bit, when she came home, was difficult because it was trying to manage things. I think vicars are a bit like mothers in a way. Your place is usually in the wrong and you usually feel guilty for all that you haven't done, rather than feel pleased with the things you have achieved. So you tend to have a negative outlook on your own performance. And certainly that grabbed me when she first came home because I said, 'look, I'm going to work the mornings, I'm not doing any more evening meetings.' And I delegated other people. I was governor of three schools - although I had already given the governorship of one of the schools to the curate - and just covered when I could.

It was a question always of feeling guilty I suppose in that year before I retired, that I wasn't being a good carer and wasn't being a good vicar either. I don't think my faith was enhanced in that time, apart from that it was great the number of people who would come and help, and say, 'I'll come and sit with Heather if you want to do this funeral this afternoon or go off and doing something'.

I think people very quickly got used to how Heather was. People would come on a Sunday morning. With six churches the way we did it, quite often I would do two or three services. I'd start at one end of the parish at 8 o'clock, then a 9 o'clock and then a 10.30. I would get up; get her meds into her, get her a cup of tea, come back after one service; give her a bowl of breakfast cereal and start getting her dressed, and then zip off to the next one. So some of it was quite tiring physically.

I was all right as a cook. I suppose I'm pretty much the same now. What I find now is the boredom of having to cook; the housewife bit. I suppose all the time I've been a vicar, because I was the one resident at home, I did most of the shopping; I did most of the cooking in the evening. I'd have a sandwich at lunch while Heather was a Mrs Two Dinners. She'd have a cooked lunch at school and then expect another one when she came home!

Now it's particularly about looking at her weight; watching and being very aware how much more weight she's put on. Since the stroke she's put on five stone, which is getting towards Type 1 Diabetes and I'm thinking 'oh boy'. It's being the food police and that's tough, not good for relationship!

We haven't really found any adaptations necessary, only minor ones. I realized, because of mobility things, we had to have a walk-in shower, so what we'd planned as a much smaller bathroom; we switched around. And I've put in several handrails.

Giving counsel to people in this situation? I'd be very careful in what I said at all! A colleague of mine, three months before Heather had her stroke, his wife had a stroke as well, and she went to Frenchay. They didn't give her a craniectomy and after two and half weeks she died. So, I'm aware of that.

As a vicar I've never sold people places in paradise, and all that kind of thing. It's just not on. And similarly I'd be very cautious about anything I said to anyone else, because each person responds so differently to a stroke. I would probably just say 'have courage; keep your pecker up; keep going; keep responding; don't give up.' I wouldn't say, 'oh it will all be better in a couple of weeks', because sometimes it just isn't.

I always remember the late Bishop Eric who was in my last parish. His wife had a stroke just as we were coming into Coleford. I saw her in hospital and she'd lost her speech centre. But she was still quite bright. She was not mobile. Bless him, he used to go and see her every day; and sit with her more or less the whole day; read her the newspaper. He would have this conversation with her, and all she could do was go 'bbbbbb'. But you could tell by the intonation of her voice when you really listened, that she was approving or disapproving. I walked in one day with shorts on – it was a hot day – and she went 'oooobbbbb', and I knew, oh dear, I should have worn long trousers.

JOHN DAVIS

John is a friend who lives just up the hill from me in coastal Dorset. When Annie and I first came here house hunting, we called into John's hotel for a cream tea: just two hundred yards from the seashore. Months later, John had to give up the hotel after his stroke and now uses a walking frame to get around. Previously he had enjoyed walking his guests over nearby beauty spot Golden Cap as a delightful excursion before Sunday lunch. Here is John's story:

At the age of seventeen, doing National Service, I volunteered to go to Germany. Because they didn't know what to do with me, they put me in what they called the Work Study Unit, which was about twelve blokes going around Germany, mainly in private cars belonging to the officers, to various projects authorised by the Air Ministry. Things like stock management.

The biggest project we did was on the Hunter aircraft turn-round. We clocked all the activity that went on when they landed, until they took off again. Like re-arming, refuelling; and checking the instruments; replenishing the camera film. Originally they had teams of six or seven different technicians swarming over the thing. Our job was to reduce that figure. Originally it took them thirteen minutes to get them airborne again, so the Air Ministry was very concerned to make it very much shorter. We recorded every activity; had little symbols for various activities.

In the end we got it down to about seven minutes. We even hit the front page of the Daily Telegraph. We did it by sharing the various mechanics; not keeping strictly to their skill. We even got the pilot ticking a checklist, though they weren't very happy about it.

One of the things we did was organise a skiffle group, the four of us, and we used to perform at the camp cinemas around Germany, which was very popular at the time - Lonnie Donegan was all the rage. We didn't do anything very special; in fact it was rubbish. I used to play the harmonica, which I was reasonably good at. We had the tea chest, the guitarist, the washboard – all the traditional stuff for skiffle. We used to get a lot of parties in the officers' mess, Christmas time. It was all part of the good life out there.

When I came out of the Air Force after two years National Service it was all a bit flat. I had a job with WH Smith at the time, which I started when I left school, on the bookstall in Bath. I didn't want to do that because life had been so exciting. I wrote to head office asking if they had anything in Organisation and Methods. They said 'oh yes, we're just starting a project on retail methods, you're welcome to come and join the team in London'.

I got a train to London fairly soon and never went back to the bookstall. I found myself some digs and went to work at head office; on a project about the paperwork for shops to order books. I devised various things, like a scheme that combined the order with a tear-off slip that was stuck in the books sent.

After about three years I went on to various jobs in Organisation and Methods for more money. By then I was living with Peter, my mate from Bath, in a lovely cottage pied a terre in Wimbledon, and after that I got a flat in Wimbledon. But I thought O and M was a bit too broad a spectrum. In the early sixties people were just beginning to think of computers. Joe Lyons the catering people had looked round the world for a computer suitable for customer management, but couldn't find anything, so they started a computer company of their own, which they called Leo (Lyons Electronic Office).

I saw an advert in The Economist from Southalls Birmingham, who had bought one of these Leo computers. They wanted staff to look after that. So I joined them as a systems man, and in the end I became the golden balls future boy from the group board down for what I did. I was twenty-six, and I think we were expecting our first child then. This was the beginning of my life in computers.

I was there about ten years, but got more ambitious for more money. I left Sanaco Computer Services, as it had become by then, and the rest of my working life is really about Fletcher Computer Services, a company on the other side of Birmingham that wanted to revitalise their business. I started by sorting out the computer chaos, was there for about twenty-five years and I ended up holding a hundred per cent of the shares by a long and circuitous route.

They were trying to run this bureau at a profit, but doing all the old-fashioned applications that didn't make money. It was owned by a merchant bank and they sent one of the accountants from another company they had closed down, and he joined the company as Financial Director.

After a year or so we made a move towards share ownership, and he devised a deal where we bought the company from the bank, with one of the bank's directors. We were one-third owners each. We then bought out the bank man, and then sadly Desmond died suddenly. I was then co-owner with his new young wife, until we came to an arrangement, and I was sole shareowner. We went from strength to strength, until in 1995 I sold the company, and in 1998 bought a hotel in Dorset.

I was sixty-two, and my second wife who is younger had always been in catering: a bit of a management character in Berni Inns. We had a young daughter. It was really an investment on my wife's part; I was retired really, but I still got involved.

We had a nice bar built because a bar is the place everyone gets to meet in a hotel. Indeed, crowds of people came down to the bar before dinner. Caroline ran the place really: the office, the billing, and did the menus. We upgraded the feel of the place quite a lot. It was all very pleasant; it was all going very well - until I had my stroke in 2003. And when the stroke came along, bang, that was it.

I had a lot of jobs at the hotel. I used to do all the gardens, everything to do with the drinks, the wines, so my wife didn't have to worry about any of that. I used to do quite a lot of shopping before the good times when all the suppliers delivered to the hotels and catering establishments. I used to make sure things like the oil lamps on the table were always ready for use. But when I had the stroke I couldn't do anything.

I went to the doctor because I was very short of breath, and he gave me some antibiotics that didn't seem to do anything. The shortage of breath got worse and worse and I had to go into Dorchester hospital because I could hardly breathe. It was pneumonia really. There was no sign of a stroke at this point.

What they thought had happened was that being in a bar I used to meet all sorts of people who had travelled all over the world; and they thought I'd caught a bug from one of them from the Far East. Because there was a thing called SARS around, they thought it was something like that.

I wouldn't respond to any of the drugs they were giving me. They could only treat me with broad spectrum ones anyway as they didn't know what it was - which were not as strong as normal ones. In the end the breathing got so bad they decided to put me on a breathing machine with all the dials and knobs to control the oxygen: also because I wouldn't tolerate an oxygen mask on my face all the time. I found it much too inconvenient, or too uncomfortable – I kept ripping it off.

I think I was short of supply on the oxygen some time; obviously a knob the nurse turned to get it right. I can't prove it but I think my stroke was caused through lack of oxygen. So it wasn't the primary cause I was in hospital; it was a secondary thing that happened during the stay. But because they were in the process of saving my life I decided not to sue them; not to make any fuss about it. If they hadn't put me on this breathing machine I probably would have copped it; an induced coma so there wouldn't be any stress on my body.

I was quite ill. I had things like sepsis, all the things going round at the time. And they even put me in isolation at one point, because they thought I'd got this hospital virus. I don't think my little child was impressed with all that. The most she knew of me when she was little was that I was ill, in hospital.

Eventually my body diagnosed what this was exactly, which was very clever of it, and immediately dealt with it, and in about two days. Amazing. With all the knowledge the path lab had, and all the tests on my blood, they didn't have a bloody clue. But my system finally got hold of it and killed it in two days.

Fortunately my wife was there when I became conscious again, and woke to friendly surroundings. Meantime my daughter who was about four had visited me several times with my wife, and she seemed to take it all in her stride, even though she was very young. She made sure I had something to read, like a newspaper. Sometimes she would even read the headlines to me.

The effects of the stroke were, I couldn't move at first, totally immobilised. I did physiotherapy lying in the bed. They had no choice but to send me home again. My mobility had improved quite a lot by then. One of the best things I did when I first came out of hospital was some therapy at home. A lady came to the house twice a week and she tried to get me to do basic exercises; standing, moving my legs and all that. That went on for a year probably, and then she recommended I went on to this thing called Pulse, approved by the doctors, which means 'Prescribed Use of Leisure and Sports Equipment'.

I don't know why more people don't do it, because it involved a six-week course at a gymnasium locally – I went to Axminster, where they have a health expert in charge. They test you on a walking machine to see what you can do and prescribe a series of exercises for you; treadmill or whatever. So I went on to this and within about two weeks all the movement in my legs and all the muscles in my legs returned back to normal. Amazing recovery, because my legs were like spindles, no muscles at all. Suddenly, in about two weeks my muscular power came back, and I was able to walk with the support of a frame very easily, and I could perform fairly normally once I got to my feet on the frame.

I've since met one or two other people who have done that and they've said the same; it's brilliant. The muscles heal very quickly, but it left me with a problem down my left-hand side, left hand and left leg – which are pretty uncontrollable. It took away my balance completely, so I shall always need some sort of walking aid, which I suppose will always be the case since it's now thirteen years since the stroke. But it's certainly improved immensely since then.

Otherwise everything else seems all right, thank God; cross everything. My mental faculties seem to be untouched. My speech isn't as it normally was, but not unreasonably so. Not quite so articulate as I used to be perhaps – perhaps a bit too loud-mouthed! You sort of get lazy without realising it.

I think I've been reasonably fortunate really. It could have been a lot worse. When you see some of these people whose brain gets completely addled. You've got to manage things. Because I was a left-handed writer and the stroke affected my left-hand side, I had to learn to write right-handed. I had a lady who came to the house. She used to teach me how to write, and she was very patient with me, because it was very, very difficult. But she persisted with me and I could manage to write sufficiently to cope with everyday things.

I wouldn't say I could write a long letter, although I did practise; I started writing my life story, which I got quite a long way with. I think I got about twenty pages; then I got fed up with it! Now I can just about make myself understood, but cheques are just a scribble, but it's the same scribble and it seems to get accepted by the banks and people. But when I try to do my signature I can't do that at all, because it's totally a left-handed signature. The advice I'd give to other stroke people is 'whatever you've got left use it or you'll lose it. Keep what you have got active'.

My wife and I had had four happy years running the hotel, because we seemed very complementary. After the stroke she seemed to be very stoical. She realised, of course, what a hole it would be in the running of the hotel because she would have to take over all the things I'd been doing. But she recruited a barman and found a nice contractor for the gardening, the lawns. Employing odd people here and there, she managed to cope quite well. She was very organised on the computer, using a proprietary hotel management system, which I could operate under great difficulty if I had to.

She had been the guts of the organisation while I was doing the sociable part of it, but because of my lack of mobility I never did anything again. With me out of the way it all had to be done by other people. The net result was two things; the additional stress upon her. And a slight reduction in profits because of the staff and facilities that had to be employed. That wasn't very good really, but it wasn't disastrous and she successfully ran the hotel for another ten years or so. She made some good decisions, like moving over from full catering to bed and breakfast, which was more profitable because staff costs far less.

It also meant she had more time off so it was a little more relaxing. I suppose the answer to how it changed anything about our relationship, is that we've always been fairly independent people. For example, we weren't the sort of couple who sat around watching television together all night; we've never done that. If she wanted to watch something, she would watch it, and if I wanted to watch something else, I would catch that. And we'd stand in for each other in the hotel.

At lunchtime I often used to cook the lunch, so that didn't happen any more. We had our daughter to worry about, which we didn't have in the early days. Caroline has always said my daughter didn't have sleepless nights, so didn't have anxieties about it, which was amazing. But she was a happy little girl when I started to show signs of life and come round a bit.

After the ten years my wife determined to get a good buyer for the hotel, and in the end we made our price and made a profit on it. In the meantime we had built a very nice house on the old car park of the hotel. Since we didn't need to buy that land and just had building costs; it was a good asset to have; its value now is much higher.

From the financial point of view things haven't turned out too badly. When I first came out of hospital, which was about two or three months after I went in, Caroline thought I'd be in a wheelchair all the time, which I was initially, and she thought the access in the hotel would not be as good as it ought to be for me. First of all she bought a house, just opposite the flat I'm in now, which was very nice, but was too large for us really. We had that for two years and she sold it.

After that, she decided to get me a flat, and one came up the road from here. It was quite a largish two bedroom flat, but a bit difficult for access. Now I'm in another flat on the ground floor and much more accessible. Caroline seized the opportunity to get a lease on this flat. Caroline went to live with my daughter in the house we built on the hotel car park, and we decided to have it converted to be more suitable for me, with my own lounge, bedroom and bathroom; a walk-in, non-slip shower like here.

But once she got her hands on the architect she decided to have other things done, so the date for when I might move back into the house has gone back and back and back. But I'm quite relaxed about that. There are certainly no problems or animosity between Caroline and I at all. We've always had a very good relationship, and if anything I think the stroke and its aftermath has probably strengthened that relationship.

While we weren't dependent on each other in any particular sense, we relied on each other to run the hotel together. Now I'm disabled I certainly need her to help me as a carer, but she's very capable of being a carer. Being twenty-three years younger, she is much more energetic in being able to take care of me, than I would be married to someone of my own age. She does all the shopping I need, and she's very good at anticipating what I require; sometimes before I even know I need it.

For instance, one day she turned up with two or three packets of my favourite cornflakes; and I saw them in her arms and said, 'why have you brought those?' She said, 'you need them'. Sure enough I had about a spoonful left. In fact I think my diet has improved since I got laid up. I eat a lot more fruit. I only have one meal a day, sometime in the afternoon.

Caroline does all the banking on-line now, standing orders – like for the flat rent – and most things now: my Wiltshire Farm Foods: a whole month's supply. They are fantastic and not that expensive. She looks after all the financial side of things; which she always did, and any papers that come to me I pass them on to her so she can understand them.

I was philosophical about it really, especially when I got the power of my limbs back. I thought that was very good indeed. And it's not really been a serious problem except I'm not very mobile and can't get about much; especially because at the moment my scooter has to be kept down the road a bit, because there's no room here. I used to be able to go to the shops or hairdressers on my scooter, but I can't get to it now. The only way is to get a lift down to the garage by my wife. I don't even know if the battery's charged at the moment. I've temporarily abandoned that.

As I say Caroline and I were always fairly independent socially. I'm not in a rush to go back to the house, I've got my computer and that amuses me a lot. I say I keep my brain active deliberately. I do a lot of Scrabble on line. I don't get tired. I stay up late and if there's a late film I watch that until one or two in the morning; doesn't bother me at all. I'm okay in the shower and toilet; I don't need any help on that. I don't even do much reading now, but if I need to I've got lots of books to read. I go to stroke club once a week – where people think I'm very jolly – I remember all their names and make a point of addressing everyone. And I go to a day centre.

But eventually I guess I will go back. I'll just hang on until all the works are finished and it's time for me to go back. All in all I'm very happy with my lot. No problem at all.

COLIN McDERMOTT

Colin's wife Ros is my cousin. She first told me of Colin's stroke when they came to stay with Annie and me in France. Ros and I were close as children, but inevitably moved apart in later years. Subsequently, I was impressed when I discovered that Ros was a Francophile, deeply involved in twinning and that she loved our part of Normandy. When they visited they told us what had happened to Colin. It's another major reason for writing this book. Here is Colin's story told mostly through Ros:

At the time we lived in a village in Nottinghamshire, and Colin had previously worked for ten years in Kuwait. We were married with three children. They were all grown up then and had left home when Colin had his stroke. He was fifty-two at the time and seemingly healthy. He hadn't been to the doctor for sixteen years, which came out later, after the event. Apparently the doctor had said to him sixteen years previously, that he needed him to go away, lose weight and make another appointment.

Sixteen years on, when he had done none of those things, he began to have strange episodes. We would be out for a drink and he'd have perhaps a couple of drinks and then act as though he'd had a bottle and a half. I was actually rapidly losing patience with him and was thinking about leaving him at the time because it was getting me down.

And on the 15 June 1996 we went to a neighbour's anniversary party and after about half an hour somebody came to me and said, 'did you know Colin was drunk?' and I said 'oh, I'm not going home yet I've only just got here'. The following day, which was a Sunday, he actually drove the car and we went to fetch my mum for lunch. And then he didn't feel so well, so I took her home. We were supposed to be going out that night and while I was in the bath he came into the bathroom and talked utter gibberish really; like speaking in tongues, that's the only way I can describe it.

I got him into bed and obviously we didn't go out. I rang the locum doctor and the doctor didn't want to come out because he was watching something on the television. He said 'whatever's happened has happened, so just leave him in bed.' At 10 o'clock when I couldn't get any sense at all from Colin I insisted the doctor came out, which he did. He said 'something has happened, but I don't know what. I'll leave a letter here for your doctor; make an appointment with your GP as soon as you can.'

On reflection, that doctor needed a kick in the teeth, but Colin was only fifty-two and it never occurred to me that it could possibly be a stroke. Colin had not told me any of his symptoms and that the previous Saturday – which I didn't find out until long after the stroke and he'd got back to speaking again – he'd actually had an out of body experience. He's just not the sort of man to do that.

It was when we were having a coffee morning for the twinning association and he was sitting in our village centre. He said that all of a sudden he was above himself, looking down. That was before the stroke, so obviously it was forty-eight hours coming. With hindsight I would have dialled 999, but I didn't know what was going on.

Colin: Let's go back though. While I was in the Middle East I played squash every day, so I was in a hot climate, which thinned the blood, and I took salt tablets as well. So my blood was thin and presumably that was okay while out there. But when I came back to this country my blood thickened up because I'd stopped taking salt tablets in the cold climate. It raised the blood pressure that caused the stroke. There was no indication of that, because I was quite fit.

Ros: On the Monday I tried to make an appointment but I couldn't get one until the Tuesday. So Colin didn't get any attention until after the Tuesday, and just stayed in bed. It's so horrific when I think about it now.

Our GP thought it was a stroke and Colin at that time had some private health insurance, so we went for him to have a brain scan. Obviously from the scan they could tell that he'd had a stroke and he'd had a hemorrhage behind one eye. Lots of things came out of that, but at no point did he go into hospital.

We didn't get any help; nobody was interested really. I felt dumped in it, and I just got him back to health the best way I could. He could speak hardly at all; his right side was affected, and the left side of his brain; so he'd lost a lot of memory and he kept falling over. He started on Warfarin straight away, prescribed by the GP, who was very kind and thoughtful – more than anybody really. We just plodded on with it after that.

I was thinking I've got to do something about this because there's only me who can sort him out. I tried the British Heart Foundation and they suggested I got some of their booklets. I tried Headway, which was in Nottingham, for people with brain problems, but they weren't interested because he hadn't had a motorbike accident. And he was too young for old people's places.

We were offered nothing at all, so we did all the therapy at home. He didn't talk at all after the stroke. We started by putting names on all the items like the fridge, so he could point if he wanted anything, and gradually his speech came back. We did it by being very, very patient with him, and showing him things and saying 'what's this?' He wouldn't answer the phone or anything; he'd lost confidence entirely. I had to get a mobile so that if anybody rang home he could listen to the message and then he could call and tell me.

I was having to work and leave Colin at home - I had to carry on working until three years ago. I had my parents up here as well. My dad had got dementia and my mum had cancer, so I just took it all on board. When I think about it now I don't know how I got through it really.

Gradually I got Colin to make a cake, and that was how I started him back on doing things. He couldn't do anything else to start with, and that was my way of giving him confidence and independence. I gave him a simple recipe and left him to it.

Colin: I think you need to do something, like the cooking. I started with cakes, and then I started to get the dinner ready. Got to do something to keep yourself occupied. If you've been someone who has been quite active their whole life, and then have to be sedentary, it makes a hell of a difference. You need to do something.

Ros: Eventually Colin was able to speak, and he had to have driving lessons again. I had to take him to Derby to go on a simulated driving course. Nobody would actually say whether he could go on the road or not, but eventually they said he could, and after fourteen months he went back to work. I don't think he should have with hindsight.

I think that after he went back to work, in late 1997, it wasn't long before he was having what I now know were several TIAs. One day I came home and his shirt was thrown on the bed, covered in blood. Apparently he'd gone to one of the sites – he was a planning engineer – and he'd fallen flat on his face. They had let him get back in the car and drive home from Leeds, which was about an hour and a half from here. He got back here, changed his clothes, and went back to work! He was so affected he didn't think that was the wrong thing to do. That's one of the things that was lacking; he hadn't got any common sense, and nobody helped him.

And then in 1999 he was coming home from work, and I think he had another TIA. He smashed into a parked car - fortunately in our village, opposite the doctors' surgery. Someone fetched me – a nineteen year old lad who lived quite close by – and said, 'Ros I think Colin's had another stroke; he's had an accident.' I went to sort it out and Colin was not making a lot of sense, so I sent him over to the doctors. They didn't know what to do with him.

He had chest pains then, and it went on for about ten days and that's when, 9 September 1999, he had nine cardiac arrests. We'd gone for a walk, and he said he didn't think he could get home. So I ran home, got the car, went and picked him up. He said I'm just going to lie down, and I felt, I'm just on this, and phoned 999.

I don't think Colin remembers the paramedic coming. The driver with Paul the paramedic said, 'oh he'll be all right', but Paul took one look at him and got him in the ambulance. He had a massive heart attack in the ambulance outside our house. The paramedics told me to drop everything and get in the ambulance. 'We don't know if we'll get there, we've used everything.' So I got in the ambulance and a neighbour came with me, thank goodness.

He had nine more cardiac arrests when he got to the hospital, which really blew the whole thing again, because of lack of oxygen. We got to Kingsmill hospital and Betty and I were shown into a room. After about fifteen minutes a nurse knelt in front of me, and I thought 'this isn't good.' She said, 'we can't keep resuscitating your husband because he's only breathing himself for a couple of minutes at a time. We can't do it any more'.

But the next thing I knew he was okay, and they took him up to the ward. Colin is a quiet man - and he says even less now - but he kept shouting between every bout of resuscitation, which is why they kept going. But they didn't expect him to live through the night. The next morning the paramedics and the registrar from the night before, came to see if he was still there. That was when the children came; they were all there. That was the first time I'd asked for help. Colin doesn't remember any of it, but he's still here seventeen years later.

Colin's balance isn't really very good. We have tried bikes, but we are at walking level at the moment. We walk well, as long it's at his pace, and we can stop and rest. 'As long as the footpaths are pretty level,' says Colin. 'It's when they get uneven I have problems, because your foot tips and then you are leaning over.'

He's not been allowed to drive – and he used to do all the driving when we went anywhere. Now he likes to play with the Satnav, so that keeps him off my case! I'm fine with the driving, but we do less now. I'm seventy and Colin's seventy-one, and I have less energy now.

Colin: So we drive a hundred and fifty miles per day, and then we rest. Like when we went to France this year, we drove to Ashford and stayed in a hotel. And then we wake up in the morning and go across and drive half way down to where we're going in the Loire Valley. And rest.

Ros: That's worked really well, but Colin's energy levels are quite low, aren't they, and when we're away we tend to go out fairly early in the morning and come home soon after lunch and let him rest. Then we can maybe have a walk in the evening. But days out are quite difficult.

Colin: Yes, we have to be very selective on where we go for days out. We went to see a relative at the Tower of London and it nearly killed me! I didn't realise there were so many steps and being out all day and then walking up and down steps; even down is as bad as going up.

Ros: Colin's speech is good now, but he wouldn't answer the phone for a long time; you don't like it now, do you? He's still not good on the phone, still gets muddled. He can't think ahead and I find he makes silly decisions sometimes. He will just put the phone down if he gets muddled.

I have never resented it, but I sometimes think I'm never going to be able to go where I want to go, if you know what I mean. I do things on my own when I can; aquafit, and French conversation every week, and Colin has never minded me going out doing things.

Because of the problems, I like quite a lot of noise and he doesn't. I would enjoy a musical but he wouldn't. So I've been to Jersey Boys, for example. We have tried the other end of the scale, like Shakespeare, but he just cannot understand it.

The children have always been supportive but at the time they were a hundred miles from our home. Colin used to be very placid but we do have ups and downs now. The constant trying to understand what he means if he comes out with tomatoes when he means bananas. Things are misremembered all the time. He says he knows what he wants to say, but something else comes out of his mouth. But it comes and goes. I said to him this morning, you're remembering more than I am. He's coming out with more things now. And I said to him 'we're a good pair'!

I can't ever switch off really. I'm now taking Amitriptyline because I wasn't sleeping at all. I hadn't had a decent night's sleep for I don't know how long, and it has affected my digestion; I can't eat this that and the other. But we wake up in the morning thinking what are we going to do; what have we got to do; is there any rush? Just normal really.

As a partner you've got to be very patient, and I do lose my patience sometimes. In fact I lost my patience with him yesterday, and slammed out of the house saying 'I'm off now'! You've got to support without letting them know you're supporting, and not expect anything from them. And that's really hard when you're with someone who's been independent. And it's hard for them as well.

You have to laugh about it when things go pear-shaped. Like we stayed in a self-catering cottage this year, and the first thing, Colin broke the tin opener; it came apart in his hand. The second thing: he put on the wrong hotplate and boiled the oven glove. Unfortunately the alarm didn't go off and there were flames coming off the oven glove before I managed to rescue it. The third thing; he left a CD in the CD player and we came away with just the sleeve.

You have to keep your sense of humour!

DAVE COTTRELL

Dave is the volunteer group coordinator of 'Different Strokes', Dorset, which offers support for younger stroke survivors in Bournemouth, Christchurch, Poole and surrounding areas. He lives with his wife Carole in a delightful apartment close to the sea in Bournemouth where I visited them. They are committed Christians and feel their faith has sustained them through Dave's stroke experience. Here is Dave's story:

I owned some properties and I did all my own maintenance and repairs; development work on these properties: decorating, electrical work, plumbing. I've always done it, all my married life I've done DIY projects, and I was very active in that. Physically I was capable of running and jumping and climbing ropes and all sorts. Of course my stroke has taken all that away, and I've given all my tools to my boys and other people and got rid of everything I used to use. I can't climb a ladder now, so...(sighs)

We'd just been on holiday in Guernsey, my wife and I. We'd come back on the ferry overnight, landed in the morning, went to bed that night. When I woke in the morning we were just chatting, thinking of getting up, and I said to my wife 'my foot's going numb; oh, my leg's going numb', and it went all the way up the left side of my body. And I said to her 'I think I'm having a stroke'. I said, 'I need to get to the toilet', and I couldn't get out of bed. And when I did manage to sit on the edge of the bed I couldn't stand.

Initially Carole rang the surgery because it was just opening, and the surgery asked her some questions and said 'you'd better call an ambulance'. So she did. And the paramedics came and talked to me and they said, 'we think he's had a stroke, but we'll take him in and check'. So they took me into hospital; I went into A & E at Bournemouth hospital, and within a few minutes they'd whisked me into a CT scanner and checked me out, and confirmed I had had a stroke.

Carole: When I rang the hospital they said it was a stroke, and even though you think it might be, when it's actually said to you it's a shock. I had friends and family who thought I coped with it quite well. The way I looked at it, had it been twelve months earlier I'd have had three disabled people to look after, because I still had my mum and dad living with us. If a week or ten days earlier we'd have lost our holiday, which we enjoyed.

Because Guernsey was just across the water we didn't think of taking travel insurance. We had been cliff walking there, and I thought, 'what would I have done if it had been last week! Would I have left him to find a phone - because his mobile wasn't working – or waited and hoped somebody had come along?' So I was grateful it happened where we could cope with the situation. (We also found out later he would have been taken to a hospital in Cornwall, because that was where they dealt with strokes from Guernsey. The expense would have been difficult.) Looking positively at things was the way I coped with it.

Dave: I knew it was happening to me. I was fully awake all the time. No pain; just a sensation of numbness down my left side. I must admit initially my thoughts in the hospital were, 'well that's it, I'm going to be in a wheelchair for the rest of my life'. Within a day or so they had me out of bed, as they do in hospital these days, and put me in a wheelchair and I was scooting myself around the ward myself. I was quite adept at doing it too! I used to get myself down into the television area of the ward and watch the TV in the evenings, and I was always the last one up. They would tell me, 'you've got to go to bed now'.

I couldn't walk on my own at all. I had to have someone to support me to walk. I tried but it wasn't possible. Then they held me in the middle of my back to allow me to walk in the ward, and that was the beginnings of recovery I guess. My wife and my family who came to visit me were amazed at the progress I seemed to be making in the first few days.

Carole: I'd known people with strokes but not on a day–to-day basis. When I went to see Dave he couldn't sit on his own, and the only way was to put him in a wheelchair or armchair so he could hold himself there. He had no sense of gravity. But he improved dramatically.

Two weekends later we had something on at church and I asked if he could come home for that weekend. They said it was too early; I wouldn't be able to cope. But they said if I could come in tomorrow morning, before visiting, they would give me an hour and show me how to walk with him, as he still wasn't walking on his own. The next day he was already walking. They didn't want to give him a walking aid as they felt he would become reliant on it.

Dave: Initially I said I feel I can go home, and they said I could go home for the weekend. But it didn't happen. They wanted to look at the home to make sure I'd be safe, and there was someone who could go home with me on the Friday. But when they saw the facilities in my home, because we'd already had my wife's parents with us for a few years who were elderly and needing a chairlift and wet-room, they could see we were well set-up. So they said I could stay there.

Carole: We had somebody come in. They would take him out and walk with him: past two houses and bring him back; then three houses the next day. And when I started taking Dave out I would drive very close to the supermarket so we could go in and we'd pick up a trolley and he could use that as his walking aid. He would do a couple of aisles then I'd have to take him out to the car. But it got to the stage we could park across the car park. We improved it by doing things like that.

I did encourage him. What we did a lot of - which I got bored with but we needed to do it – I collected around the house about ten items: different pieces of fabric, a kitchen sponge, something harsh, something wrinkly, a piece of velvet, a hair brush and used to rub his leg and foot, to encourage the movement back.

We did that for months, almost on a daily basis. He had to encourage me to do it and I had to encourage him on other things. We worked together. I was at the stage where I was able to spend all my time with Dave. I'd just lost my mum and dad and the last of my kids was away. We could eat when we wanted to, go out when we wanted, not tied to regular meals as we had been.

Dave: I must admit I would sit in the bed, moving my hand, moving my foot, my leg, trying to make everything work, determined to try and get everything back. But it didn't happen as quickly as I wanted! That's the thing I most remember about having a stroke, it was frustrating that it didn't get better quickly.

I've since learned that you've just got to keep going from where you are, and take each day as it comes.

It was almost a year between the two strokes. The second one .... we go to church each Sunday and I wasn't feeling very well that morning, and I said to my wife I think I'm going to stay at home. We lived in a house that had three floors and up on the second floor I had what I called my office, where my computer was. I was happy going upstairs; I had no problem climbing stairs by then. (It was difficulty with the balance I had going downstairs.) I sat at my computer and as I sat there the room started spinning. I thought this is weird; I thought oh no, I'm having another stroke. I couldn't believe it.

I thought, I'm determined to let somebody know about this and I knew where my wife was. But I couldn't see my phone to dial the numbers properly – I was kind of dizzy. So I thought I would crawl downstairs to my bedside where my mobile phone was, switched on, and somebody had phoned me the day before who knew me and knew my family and where we went to church. I found that call and rang this person, a tradesman, and explained the problem and asked him to contact my wife.

Instead he rang 999 for an ambulance, but unfortunately they couldn't get in, of course, and I wasn't in a position to get downstairs by then. They spoke to me on my mobile and I said 'break the door down'. But they're not allowed to do that, they get the police to do that. The next thing I knew they were at my bedside, and apparently they had managed to fiddle a lock somehow and get in.

By the time my wife got home I'd been taken to hospital. I was scanned again and confirmed another stroke, and where it was. I was admitted to the ward again, so I knew the ropes by then, what was going to happen, roughly. As the first time, after a few days I was taken down to Christchurch rehabilitation hospital, and I made a similar kind of progression in my recovery. But by then they had a 'supportive release', where you go home and they send physiotherapists and other specialists to the home for a few days. So I was able to leave the hospital earlier than I might have done otherwise.

I was grateful to be out of the hospital, to have decent food my wife cooks. Just to be in familiar surroundings. I had these supportive people; someone came to talk about my swallow problem. As long I concentrated on swallowing I was okay – I didn't need liquids or anything, I just needed to be careful I didn't choke on things. I made sure I swallowed deliberately on one side.

One of my friends is a singing teacher and musician. I spoke to her and asked if there was anything I could do to help with my speech – which was fairly okay - but mainly my swallowing. She said 'have you tried singing?' I had at church, but she said, 'no, if you sing properly'. So she came to the house and asked me to sing. From then on I used to sing a bit more robustly. It has helped. I'm not sure if it's helped my speaking. It probably has, but I haven't noticed. I still mix my words up sometimes, but not very much.

I think my memory is all right, but my wife tells me I forget things. Maybe I do, but I don't notice it. It hasn't been a problem for me personally. I look at other people, and think, well, I shouldn't complain at all.

But it's me. I've got this experience; nobody else has. And it's how I feel. And even now I'm not right; I'm struggling. Every day is a challenge. I walk down the street sometimes and foolishly I look at people and think, 'you don't know what you've got'. And it's stupid, but it's how I feel sometimes: fleeting moments of self-pity. You just have to put them to one side and say 'get on with things', because you have to really, don't you?

After my stroke I was very self-indulged. I didn't really think how other people were reacting to me. I was just grateful to see them. It was wonderful to have my family to support me. But I realise now some of them went through some pretty difficult times, just looking at me and seeing how I was doing. But it was very encouraging to be told I was doing well. To the outside appearance you look as though you're fine. They don't know the inside do they. Though I do smile a lot; that helps.

Initially, when you are in hospital you are given so many different pamphlets; you're not really receptive to all that stuff at the time because you've got enough problems of your own without reading all this material. So I didn't read everything; brought it home; and probably some of it is still tucked away in an envelope somewhere. But I did get invited to some of the NHS meetings they had for clinical assessments on how things were going from their point of view. They wanted feedback.

I went to most things I was invited to. One of those events we met a couple; the wife had had a stroke and the husband was supporting her. They got talking about where they went, which was Different Strokes. It sounded very interesting and we got the details where they were meeting. I just turned up one time at St Mark's church hall in Bournemouth and asked if I could join their group. They said I could and made me very welcome, although I've since found out Different Strokes is intended for the under sixty-fives, and I was already sixty-five.

I found it very useful just talking to others who seemed to understand what I was going through, and I understood what they were going through. It was just brilliant to talk to other people with similar difficulties. Nobody's got the same problems, but it's very similar. If they've had strokes they will understand how you're feeling.

We went to those meetings from then on, and I'm now the local Dorset group coordinator. I organise the monthly meetings we have and keep in contact with the people who have given us their contact details. I email them primarily, but I do have a few phone numbers and some postal addresses for those who don't have email. I've got forty-three contacts on my list, so when I organise anything I send the invite out to those forty-three contacts. Although a few of these are NHS personnel, so the stroke-related members are about thirty-five.

Mainly the meeting is just to talk about anything coming up organised by The Stroke Association, by Different Strokes; anything, events to do with stroke. And to talk about how we feel about our recovery, and point people in the right direction if they don't know how to find the help they might need. The website has an awful lot of information and I developed a resource on my Google drive, where I've posted everything I've got, literature wise, that isn't on our Different Strokes website. So anything I show the group paper-wise they can access on Google drive.

I also run a Facebook group for Different Strokes, Dorset, although we do tend to call ourselves Stroke Survivors Dorset on the Facebook page. We have a sister group which call themselves Stroke Survivors Southampton. I have literature I've had developed. I've printed five thousand copies of this leaflet, and I've had these business cards produced, which has got both things on there. I've sent out a bunch of those leaflets, maybe a hundred copies, to doctors' surgeries in the Bournemouth postcode area.

I do other things besides the stroke group. For twelve years I was the director of a family history centre for our church. I was still doing that during my recovery. I only got released from that responsibility earlier this year. I was organising the staff to cover the shifts, help people with their research questions – though Carole is better than me at research. I'm more technical, and actually organised the network of six computers we have in the centre, and still do all of the maintenance on that now.

I was always involved in our church and still have responsibilities. I'm Sunday School President so organise the staffing of the Sunday school, the teachers. Help them with their teaching classrooms, their materials. I'm still as actively involved in things as I ever was. I think that's what's helped me a lot; to keep myself involved.

Am I the same person I was before my strokes? I haven't changed dramatically. I'm very much the same as I was. I still have my sense of humour – as much as I ever had! I get my sense of humour with my grandchildren more than anyone else.

I'm just slower, not able to do physical things like I used to. Not as energetic. I still have the desire to. I still think I might one day! As I said to my wife, if I survive long enough I think I'll get all of my faculties back. But I don't think I'm going to live that long! Everything takes so very long to improve. It's taken six years to get to this point, and I still have difficulty walking - although I think I could probably do eight or nine thousand steps in a day if I needed to. I think generally I do three or four thousand steps in a day. I go to the gym, usually three days a week: Monday, Wednesday and Friday for an hour or so: weights and other things.

Carole: One of the things we had decided to do when we retired was to walk. Before the stroke I had to increase my walking to catch up with him. But now I have to walk slowly to keep step with Dave. But mentally, and with chatting, it's not much different: just the physical ability to do things. He falls asleep more often. As a carer you have to try and understand and work with them. As well as giving encouragement you've also got to be aware of the limitations and not push beyond those. If you push too quickly you could do more damage than helping.

Dave: They say the cause of my stroke was hypertension and I have medication to keep that under control. It's well under control now. I don't feel the need to check it three times a day any more. In fact I'm thinking of asking my doctor if I can reduce my medication a bit. I've changed my diet as well, quite significantly. I don't eat any red meat, any dairy products at all. I don't have any sugar in anything, or salt. Occasionally I think I could do with some salt and have a packet of crisps. I'm used to it now and enjoy it. I've got a good appetite, but my portion sizes are slightly smaller. My weight is under control.

I volunteer on Ward 27 at Bournemouth hospital. My last visit one of the patients seemed pretty down, and I went over and asked if she'd like me to talk to her. I wear the Stroke Association shirt, because they sponsor the volunteers on the ward. I spoke with her for about ten or fifteen minutes. She was probably seventy/seventy-five; my age I guess. She was hoping to go home in a few days, and I encouraged her to keep doing all she could, to try and make improvements. I said that in my experience recovery does occur if you work at it. When I got up to leave she said 'Dave, I'll never forget you. Thank you for talking to me.' Often that's the case. People just need someone to talk to with a similar experience.

CHARLES SPENCER

A friend in France told me of Charles Spencer, a stroke survivor who was learning again to play the piano with his left hand. Charles kindly picked me up from my hotel and drove me back to his apartment in the magnificent White House in Harrogate. We sat at his kitchen table where he, and then his charming wife Katie, told me the story of his stroke experience and recovery:

I had my Stroke at fifty-four. I am now sixty-five. I was a commercial mushroom grower. My main customer was Asda supermarket. We grew eighty tons every week in Leeds, Blackpool, Selby and in the Republic of Ireland. The head office of Asda is in Leeds. We had a very good relationship with them for years, and in fact my company was the first to devote all of its production, or ninety-five per cent, to Asda. They were excellent regular payers.

But things had become very stressful in terms of a major virus that affected with devastating effect so many mushroom farms around the country. And that was the start of my stress. High blood pressure is the major cause of stroke, but mine was irregular heartbeat: atrial fibrilation. I'm not fat, and I was a regular gym-goer, but I wasn't sleeping too well and travelling twenty-seven thousand miles a year. Then I became involved in a legal dispute; a formidable opponent of the Inland Revenue, and also at the same time with former partners in the business. I was sleeping about four or five hours a night, perhaps over-exercising: first to the gym at half six. I can't believe I did all this, and perhaps drinking too much. Awful when I look back on it.

I'd been to the cardiologist two or three times in the six months before because there were times when you could see my heart beating through the shirt. We knew him socially, and after the stroke he said he didn't realise quite how stressed I was. I had got so used to dealing with stress that it became the norm. So I presented as a dicky heart and he gave me some medication. Nowadays, if you present as I did, even your GP prescribes Warfarin, or some other blood-thinning drug, before you even get to the cardiologist. Which I think is a huge advantage. I venture to suggest that if that had happened I wouldn't have had the stroke.

The actual stroke happened on a remote island in Greece, Skyros. I was talking to an English lady, a Doctor of English Literature, and seeing her afterwards she said it was the first time a man had fallen at her feet! Because apparently – it was before lunch – I threw my glass of water into the air and collapsed. When I came to, about five or ten minutes later, I was on the floor and the ambulance people hadn't arrived. It's an unbelievable feeling when you send messages down to your legs, arms, 'move', and nothing happens. All I could move was my left hand, which I needed to shield my face from the sun.

I was already aware there is a critical window of about five hours, I believe, when you can possibly reverse the effects of a blood clot. But there is only a field hospital on Skyros and waiting for the ferry for the mainland and an overnight stay in a country hospital, with an incredibly awful, bumpy ride on a stretcher by ambulance to Athens is difficult.

All the time Katie was in England. I was there on this course at the Skyros Centre - 'Living with your Heart'!* It was extraordinary because not long before my mother had died, and I was horrified when I saw her coffin lowered into the grave, I didn't feel anything. I thought this is really odd: I've got a total divorce between the head and the heart.

Katie came out. It was a tremendous shock. I had to stay three weeks because you can't fly. Then I got an infection from a dirty catheter. I was flown home after that and stayed six weeks in Harrogate hospital. Then you're let out on your own. I said I'm only fifty-four, with a super confident and helpful wife. Imagine having the same thing on your own in your seventies. I came here. What do I do now? I couldn't dress myself. I couldn't cook. I couldn't cut anything. But I understand now there is a dedicated stroke ward in Harrogate.

As regards the legal things, Katie was a non-executive director of the businesses, so she knew my former partners, the accountants, the bankers, the solicitors. Thank goodness. And that dispute was settled through arbitration. This was about three years after the stroke and I said I'd like to attend the arbitration. The Cardiologist looked at me, like being in the headmasters study, 'Mr Spencer, you've obviously no idea how close you were to death. I cannot imagine a more stressful situation than you are proposing.'

I played the piano from the age of eight. Apart from running and the gym that was my one and only hobby. I think with all the stress I would play the piano the two or three years before, but it was very repetitive. I would play the first movement of Beethoven's Moonlight Sonata over and over and over again because it was so calming.

Apparently that is very indicative of being under stress. Doing the same thing over and over. But I certainly found it immensely relaxing, and in fact there is a very nice man I've met recently in Harrogate who was a composer and teacher of harmony at Leeds College of Music, and he is transcribing the piece to be for left hand only.

Then the stroke happened and to see the piano but unable to play was irritating me, like owning a horse you can't ride. Then a friend who lived next door to the Head of Music at Bradford grammar school said they would give their eyeteeth for a piano of this quality. I thought, that's marvellous, and off it went for three or four years on long-term loan to his study. In fact the main beneficiary of that was a child prodigy of about eleven, and I like to console myself that every cloud has a silver lining.

Then, and I often think about this, why wasn't I aware that there was so much music just for the left hand? I knew there were exercises for strengthening, and I know the famous Ravel concerto for the left hand. Until you're disabled, it's shameful to say I'd given it very little thought.

It was talking to a neighbour in a village in France - he was a minister of the Scottish church, and also as it turns out an ex-member of the SAS. He didn't appear to me as sympathetic as many people were. He said, 'why aren't you playing with the left hand?' I said, 'well, it's not very satisfying'. This was a social lunch, and he appeared to be over-stepping normal boundaries, so I was quite offended. I've written just this last week to the host of that lunch thanking him, because I went back and there is loads of music. So I gave the Bradford school a nice amount of notice and the piano came back.

I couldn't wait for it to get back, but I was horrified; it had been eight years since I played. I'd given all my music away. I bought some music, and I was shocked, I couldn't read it. I couldn't work out key signatures. It was back to the drawing board. I had to learn to read again, which took the wind out of my sails. But moving here to this street I met a chap who is a barrister and very fine amateur pianist. He introduced me to another lady who is an ex-head mistress, concentrating on the piano. I went back to weekly lessons.

It's true I was so humiliated and embarrassed with the effects of this stroke. My face; I'd lost even more weight. It was six weeks after the stroke when I saw myself for the first time in the mirror, while no one else was there. It was such a shock. I'd read about an experiment with monkeys; how they'd taken a tendon from the ankle, transplanted to the limb. I went through procedures and meetings about my impaired right hand. The consultant said, 'while I'm confident of my own abilities, there's a fifty per cent chance that you could be left with no movement at all'.

Even simple things like shaking hands. I was always missing the other person's. So I took the decision to shake hands with the left hand only. But it's odd not having the use of a limb; or gross movement of the right limb; no fine-tuning. But I had no feeling at all down the right side until just two years ago, which meant always bumping into people and unaware: those mini embarrassments and minor shocks at cocktail parties.

But two years ago we met a lady in France who lived in Denmark. She was an anaesthetist. Her daughter was ill and she had taken her for treatment to China for six months, and while there learned about acupuncture. She was confused why I had made such progress but hadn't had the feeling return. She gave me ten days daily acupuncture - one photograph Katie took of me where I had thirty-seven needles in! Gradually the feeling returned and that's been a marvellous restoration. I'm always in her debt.

I could write with my left hand but only basically, and with the computer there isn't the need. At a recent course I was awarded an amanuensis, which was marvellous and allowed me to concentrate with the lady doing the notes, which I could read at leisure.

One of the most annoying things is this habit of inverting things. I always say the opposite. So when the nurse at the surgery said, 'remind me how old you are', when I was fifty-nine, and I said ninety-five. I was telling that story to a man who runs a stroke group here in Harrogate. He'd been an accountant in Leeds. And he said, 'you think that's embarrassing Charles'. He was seventy at the time, and he said someone asked him how old he was and he said seven!

Immediately after the stroke I was lucky to have Katie oversee all correspondence concerning the business. On one occasion she caught a payment where I had reversed the figures to the client's huge advantage!

But the main thing I'd like to say is learning to accept dependency. The chap at Stroke Club - a man of Indian extraction, an American citizen now, very fit, and big on meditation and yoga, who had a surprising stroke at the age of seventy – agrees. He said the challenges of learning to accept the dependency. Particularly for people who were pretty senior in our professions, it's doubly hard. But it's amazing how many people turn out only too pleased to help you, in restaurants and shops.

Katie says my walking is different from day to day, and she's always saying 'pick up your right foot' or whatever. And I can't see any rhyme or reason why it changes from day to day.

There was a book I read after about three years. At first I thought it was the most macabre title written by a Californian doctor or dentist who had suffered a stroke. He'd titled his book 'A Stroke of Luck'. That's precisely what I didn't think it was, but I'm accepting that. I'm more at ease with myself than I was. I was always chasing rainbows; I could never have enough money, the more money I had the more I spent. I was chasing my tail. I would never have had the satisfaction of doing what I'm doing on the piano and raising money. It's hard to think that such a dire strait leads into much calmer waters.

That book is a tremendous challenge for a stroke person. The second challenge is there is so much medically, and so many devices to help you do this, or for speech. But only now starting to address the psychological impact. It's a major shock: an inner state of shock. Not just you but for your partner for months and years afterwards.

Katie says

At the time of the stroke I had been to Skyros once. They do creative writing courses and also therapeutic courses. Charles had finished his history of art degree at York University; had given in his dissertation and he wanted to go for a break. I was finishing a Masters down at Sussex: creative writing and personal development.

What an irony to chose 'Living with your heart'. He found himself in a group with some people seriously emotionally disturbed. One woman he told me about would say, 'am I going to be alive at the end of the day, am I going to kill myself?' Towards the end of the first week he realised he couldn't keep quiet much longer; he would have to start talking about himself; and he said 'my heart's all over the place Kate'. The next day he had his stroke. As he said he had pressures at work, but that was the actual trigger.

First off, it's almost impossible to process. I remember friends of mine were picking me up to go to a garden party down the road. I had a call just as we were about to go. Luckily there was a doctor there, and she said Charles has just had a stroke. They'll be taking him to Athens. My friends left and then came back, and in the meantime I tried to go onto the computer to look at flights, but I couldn't do anything. I couldn't make my mind work, and when they came back my friend's husband Johnny said 'Nicky I think you're going to have to go with Kate', so she booked the flights, and somehow I packed.

It was awful, I felt I couldn't take it on board at all. We flew out to Athens and were looked after very well by the Skyros network in Athens, who were understandably enormously good at dealing with that sort of work, and put up in a hotel next door. It was strange seeing Charles because he looked so well. He was tanned, and he was sitting there looking fine, but he could only really say yes or no.

My father had had two strokes in his early sixties so I knew what to expect. Although he didn't lose any motor skills, he did lose his speech, and he said later, do remember Kate, I could understand everything you were saying, I just couldn't communicate back to you. So I had this knowledge, when I saw Charles, to say I may not be able to understand everything you're saying, but what you do say I will hear and I do know you will be understanding me. That was fantastic to know that.

It was very distressing for me, and obviously enormously distressing for him to be abroad where he felt he wasn't being understood anyway, and there was a foreign language around. Totally disorientating. He was in a ward with people recovering from cataract operations and these lovely Greek ladies were staying with their husbands and sleeping under their beds. Charles couldn't understand why I wasn't sleeping under his bed!

Also he had this depressing prison-type view except one amazing ray of sunshine, and this fantastic guy called Stylianos. He was a drama therapist who wore a pendant with a shank of silver with a question mark (most people there wore crosses). He was totally open, plus fluent in English, to supporting anything Charles needed. He would come and talk to him every day, and he talked him down from a headache one day, thinking it was going to be another stroke.

He said to both of us. 'We don't know why people have strokes at all; we can work out physically, but we don't always know emotionally what causes them. We do know quite a bit about various things for recovery and it's very important you're not stressed at all. And very important you are positive about what you want to do, how you want to live'.

We kept those things in our minds all the time and acted on them. We'd had this strategic discussion on how we were going to handle the difficulties around the business, so I knew, and could say this is what I'm going to do, this is right isn't it? I was given power of attorney and represented us in the various meetings.

I was pretty desperate, because I knew when I was out in Greece that he could have another stroke. I know it's quite common. I wrote the whole time. I had a journal with me and I wrote, wrote about my feelings. I couldn't think in the future very much, and when I came back I had lots of things like insurance papers, and although I'm a strong admin person I couldn't deal with it for two months or so. Bills came in but I couldn't look at them. I thought I have to totally concentrate on Charles.

I had to organise things, like another rail on the stairs, so he could go down on the left hand side; all the practical things I could deal with. When he was in Harrogate hospital he didn't like the food very much and I was cooking for him and bringing it in. I was trying to make everything as good as possible but it was all very much in the moment. I couldn't really see where we were going.

Two weeks on he got the results of his History of Art, and he got a First, but meanwhile he was completely dyslexic. He couldn't write anything; he couldn't read; he could hardly speak. Then came down with some terrible MRSA bug.

We had this guy, neurologist and I remember just after this, he came into the room, a bit careworn; his collar was worn. He sat on the end of the bed and said; 'you've had a serious stroke Charles; don't expect too much. Don't think you're going to get everything back'. We both knew he was implying the piano, because he knew Charles. He left the room, and even though Charles was dyslexic and aphasic and the awful things one can become, we looked at each other, and I said, 'it's not going to be like that is it?' And Charles said, 'no'. And from that moment on we decided, both of us - in a weird sort of spiritual communication almost - that it was going to be a positive recovery.

The one thing I knew I'd need to do. It was the end of my first year of the Masters, I knew I was going to keep doing that because I thought it would be a supportive lifeline for me. Although I had to ask for extra time for my assessment I had a couple of months and I got that all organised.

So I suppose we hunkered down and concentrated on ourselves; thinking all the time that it was going to get better. We paid for our own neuro physio, which we were lucky enough to be able to afford. We paid for extra speech therapy after the initial stuff failed. We used lots of alternative things and we were just very determined.

But the first year was quite difficult, looking back. I got fed up in the end because Charles wouldn't go to events. I said, 'you're just going to have to come with me. You must. You're not going to stay in the house'. When he did go out he had difficult things like knocking over someone's beer, but it didn't matter; he was starting to expand, and felt better about himself after a while I think.

I could see progress from day one, both in his speech, in his walking, in his ability to do things. There was quite a long time when he didn't move his right arm at all. He had the tough luck of a nurse coming, saying 'Charles, if you don't move that by the end of today, you'll never move it at all!' He was so cross, but by the end of the day he was moving his arm. She was amazing! It must be very difficult to decide you're going to act like that with someone.

Only two years after his stroke — although Charles had thought he'd go on and do further work at the Courtauld at his history of art - he actually was the first person who had had a stroke to do the MA that I had done: creative writing and personal development. And did superbly well.

He did it with an amanuensis, a friend of mine Deborah who I did my studies with, and who not only knew Charles but had actually done the course. So she was his note-taker. It was so good for Charles to have the chance himself to therapeutically write about the experiences of the stroke - and some of the other emotional sides to his life, which he'd never explored before.

We accept there are things Charles can't really handle now, so I still have to do all our finances. I did some of them before; I wasn't one of these wives where the husband did it all, but nevertheless it did tilt towards me doing everything. And I didn't really want that; it was boring. I wanted to be looked after myself; I didn't want to be the strong one all the time. So those sorts of things are very difficult for a couple I think, and have to be renegotiated and balanced. It's not always the things you see; it's the other things you don't see.

I would say to any other carer, don't believe there is any stage where improvement stops. It's continuous. I talk about brain plasticity. Charles and I are very interested in reading about all that; how the brain can develop again in different ways. I would say you may find you feel a lot closer to your partner in some ways. Charles and I have a much stronger relationship. It was good before but it's strong in a different way now. And our daughters: Charles has a girl from his first marriage and we have two.

It was Christmas, six months after Charles' stroke and I'd gone through to the kitchen to put the finishing touches to lunch. The three girls gathered round him and said, 'Daddy we've been talking about you. We've decided you're a much nicer daddy now since the stroke!' They said, 'first of all we feel you're finally listening; you're at home more. You're not always involved so much in yourself; you're more interested in what we do; you're more loving, whereas before you were so involved with your work'. It was very emotional for him and me too.

There are all sorts of things that can be good aspects. You can dwell on not walking so well or speaking so well, or you get tired. Those are obviously facets and I know there are some people who are terribly disabled and can't speak at all, so I'm not making light of that. But there are other aspects to partnership and relationships, and never give up trying to improve the disabled side either.

Charles went quite regularly to local Speakability meetings**, and then after a stage he said 'oh I think I've had enough of talking to stroke people'. And yet, interestingly, he's come full circle and is now engaging in it in a completely different way through his music. His speech recovered over the initial two years, and he wanted to see a role where you could have new meaning in your life. He had to find that; it wasn't obvious to him.

Charles: Two Christmases ago we went to a party, with carols and drinks. The person playing the piano asked me about something and I gave her a thirty-second demonstration. Then a man I'd never met before said 'you've had a stroke, haven't you, yet I've seen you playing the piano'. He runs a stroke club in North Leeds and he said he'd like me to come and play. I told him my playing was pretty basic, but my piano teacher and I went down there.

With an audience of about thirty, she spoke about the problems of teaching a brain-damaged person, how I'd progressed. I played a few pieces and then she played a nice piece of Brahms. It was a great success. They told Ilkley Stroke Club, so we've been across there. The next week Ilkley Baptist church asked me if I had any favourite hymns.

At first it was for carers or stroke-affected people, but last November it was public. It turned out very interesting. There was this lovely lady in her fifties; she does all sorts of charity work. I had told her about the playing and she thought I was joking because the fact of playing the piano left-handed. I was apprehensive, not nervous, about this concert, plus for the first time we asked people to part with money, in a public place, St Marks church.

The Lord Mayor and the Head of the Harrogate Festivals were there; as they have a large programme for disabled people in the area. The title of my piece *Inspite of Everything*, is from the French *Malgré Tout*, composed by a Mexican pianist in 1900 for his close friend (Music for the Left Hand by Paul Coker) a sculptor and keen amateur pianist, who had a major accident with his right arm. The sculpture he was working on was called *Malgré Tout*, so his friend composed this lovely tango. I'm delighted to say we raised £800 for charity and were mentioned in the Mayor's Progress Report and featured in the Harrogate Advertiser.

In fact, after the concert a ninety-year old man, a stroke survivor, came up to me and said, 'you've inspired me. I'm going to take up painting again, with the left hand'.

There has been a lot of work on the healing power of music for brain-damaged people, and there is little doubt that my speech has improved since restarting music. It's given me a purpose and restored my self-esteem.

*www.skyros.com   **www.communicationmatters.org.uk

ELIZABETH ASHMORE

I met Lizzie Ashmore on Canterbury West railway station; an unlikely place to conduct an interview, but despite the comings and goings we managed. It was fascinating to hear how she dealt with her stroke - and the extensive newspaper coverage engendered by it because of her age. With grit and determination she recovered sufficiently to return to university and set about completing her degree. Here is Lizzie's story.

I had my stroke in 2014, just over two years ago. I was studying. I was working, probably too much. I just went to Uni every day. I was overconfident. A bit too stuck up and stuff. I wouldn't say active. I walked quite a lot. The only time I'd run would be upstairs! I just used to go clubbing. I was twenty at the time, so I just followed the crowd.

I turned twenty in the October. During November, December, January I was having mini strokes, but I didn't realise. I was probably having about ten a day. The first time I thought something was wrong I was doing my makeup - just like the stroke advert - and I don't know why, but I felt a bit lopsided. I felt my face; like when you pull your face down. And I did actually joke and say 'what would you do if I had a stroke?' And my boyfriend said 'you're too young'.

I was at work one day and felt the mouth again and I kept forgetting things. My walking went a bit funny; I walked diagonally. My arm went numb; I couldn't feel it at all, and it slowly started to raise in this position permanently. It would go a bit stiff.

I went to A & E and they said it was a trapped nerve. But I had severe pins and needles down my left side and obviously that went on until I had the stroke. I didn't explain everything to A & E, but the type of stroke I had they couldn't have thrombolysed anyway.

I'd been at work all day. I got home and had a really hot bath, which didn't help. I went to bed and I was quite restless. In the middle of the night I felt a bit shaky and I tried to stand up and I just collapsed on the floor. I remember having several pins and needles down my left side to the point where it stung. I was tossing and turning all night. I remember texting my boyfriend saying 'I feel really ill, I don't feel right'.

I eventually went to sleep, because obviously my brain was shutting down, and the fatigue had started coming in. The next morning my mum ran upstairs, from what I remember, sat on the end of my bed, tried waking me up and she was asking why I wasn't at Uni. I said I'd just overslept. But my boyfriend had texted to say Lizzie hasn't texted me or been on Facebook. I said

'I can't move. I can't physically sit up', and she said 'stop joking around'. She pulled me up from my waist to sit me up straight, and I just fell to the left, just lying there.

She called my step-dad, and she dragged me to the top of my stairs (I was in the loft). My step-dad looked at me and said immediately 'she's had a stroke; call 999' - because his mum had had one. Obviously at first - I've seen pictures - my face was so drooped, and as soon as that happened I remember saying 'hospital can't cure paralysis, like there's nothing they'll be able to do.' They had to drag me down my stairs, two flights of stairs, and I was obviously quite stiff at the time. Then I went to hospital.

I saw the lights as they rushed me through. They left me in a bay until the MRI scanner was ready. All I remember is seeing my mum crying through the window - where they look at the scan. I was lying there wondering why everyone was crying over a brain. The doctor had come in and said 'you've had a stroke; you need to stay in hospital for a long time'. I just fell asleep for ages but my brain was swelling so much they thought they would have to take me to London to have it operated.

They wheeled me to the stroke ward, which was horrendous. They were older than me; it was scary, and I remember the first night in there, the woman opposite me had dementia; she kept calling to her husband. I just remember her falling on the floor, and the next morning she died; they were wheeling her away. I'd been in the top bay where you start off and all her family members had been saying 'oh she's not doing very well, she can't do this, can't do that' - to the point where I was crying. And my mum said to the nurse 'she just needs to go into another room, or be on another ward'. It took about three weeks, but they took me to a room on its own, and that's when it was fine because I had my own space.

Within the three weeks the physios had come to see me and moved my left leg up and down. Bang on the three weeks I was lifting my leg and wondering 'what's happening'. It was stiff but I remember slowing bending it. As soon as that happened I thought, 'I can learn to walk'.

My step-dad, I think he felt he'd seen his mum go through it, but for me being so young it scared him a lot. My mum wouldn't stop crying to the point where I would say 'mum, I'm going through this, not you; so stop!' I remember for weeks people sitting at my bed crying at me, and I was laying there still getting used to the fact that it had happened. I was so tired, honestly. They would cry and I would just be asleep.

I'd probably say from a young person's perspective - because apparently our brain has a higher chance of recovery - I'd just say don't treat them any different, treat them the same, and don't give them expectations; like 'your arm will come back, you'll be fine; give it a few weeks'. Don't look at them as if they are really vulnerable. Just make them feel like they are still strong. And don't ask them questions, because you don't want to talk about it at that stage. It's a blur, and where your brain is trying to connect to the blur it's a bit difficult.

In the stroke ward you have physios and occupational therapists but - no offence - they are trained to treat older people, so at that time I'd learned to start walking in that ward. They gave me this brown walking stick and I was swinging my leg. I thought 'I'm walking, I'm walking'. I remember recording it - I didn't have a splint at the time so my dropped foot was so bad I can just remember saying 'I can walk, record it, put it on Facebook'.

It makes me cry, the video. I was so happy. And then I remember my boyfriend's face, like 'no, that's disgusting'. It was literally as if I was dirt. He sat me down and said 'I'm really proud of you for doing it, but you're not walking properly', which I'm glad he said because I knew it, but I needed someone to tell me.

My mum found a rehab ward downstairs for young brain injuries, and she got me transferred after about another three weeks. That's when I probably learned. They did the whole leg placement, the way to position my foot and my leg, how to squat to get the muscle back - because you lose all feeling - how to sit up and how to stand; that was the hardest because I had Clonus (muscular spasm). I would be trying to stand up and my leg would be shaking.

They didn't really do much on my arm because the muscle tone was really bad. I couldn't open the fist. The only way to open the hand is if I bend my wrist downwards. I couldn't lift it at all, but I learned to bend it and straighten it. I've done that on my own because no one gave me physio on that (though when it's cold it gets really stiff and itchy).

I'm slow walking downstairs. I do one step at a time and my arm sticks out, so I'm more conscious. I do need to hold on, but I'm like 'no, I'm going to do it without'. They taught me that technique as well, going up one step. I felt I needed to do it faster, so now I've taught myself to skip the step. It's difficult but faster, but my knee isn't strong enough to do that going downstairs. It drops. I'll do stairs but I'll avoid them; it embarrasses me walking down.

My friends came to see me but I think it was to make me feel they were really good friends, because before we wouldn't see each other much, unless we were getting drunk! All over Facebook it was 'God, you're so strong, blah, blah.' And I think they wanted to be part of that. The Daily Mail wrote an article about me that I didn't know about, and they came in at that point.

I've only just got used to being myself. At first I would say I was depressed. I was, like, I hate myself. I wouldn't leave the house. I was in a wheelchair and my face was so bad I couldn't look at myself, I just cried. I was so depressed I'd go through 'I don't want to be alive'. And 'it's my fault'. I used to blame the lady in A & E. It was really bad. I was, effing this, effing that; she's done this to me, misjudging the trapped nerve, and if she did that to all patients then I'm scared. I slowly came out of it when I learned to walk.

I was in a wheelchair for about a month. My then boyfriend would wheel me around and people would look at me. When I went home I asked my physio if I could learn to walk outside and they said it was uneven, I'd fall over. It made me really upset and the next week I told them I didn't need them; they weren't helping me; my life needs to go on, I'm young, I need to walk. I said to mum, 'I'm going to walk to the top of the road'. I remember walking, the shortest distance for about a second and then I put my hand on this wall, I was so tired.

I kept walking around the house and my mum said 'let's venture into town with your walking stick' - the brown wooden one at the time. We walked into town, such a big achievement for me. Half an hour for a walk that now takes me about ten minutes. I was knackered but managed to walk around town. A lot of people stared, because of the brown wooden walking stick, so my mum bought me a black plastic one. After that I thought I've got to get on with it. Now I walk, not the best.

It's nice talking to people who have had the experience. Because when I first met people they'd say 'how are you, how are you doing?' and they'd look for it, whereas I'm really strong now. I went clubbing for my twenty-first, which was about nine months after the stroke, and I probably shouldn't have, because I still get it, 'oh my God, you're so strong, and I've been reading everything on your blog'. And I'd be like, 'just leave me alone'.

I didn't want to be that person, but it's probably my own fault, being in the newspaper. My boyfriend had stuck with me because right at the beginning, when I first went to hospital, my mum gave him the choice. You either stick with her or just leave now. (I only found that out about four months ago.) But after three months he said he couldn't deal with the change; and how he'd have to wheel me round in a wheelchair. He'd seen how confident I was before, and to go from that to not being confident at all, even to leave the house. And people treating me differently, and the media attention; his life became somebody else's.

I wish he'd left me on that first day because my brain was so trained to him before and after the stroke, that the first few months of splitting up I was unbelievably clingy. I'd have a go at him over nothing. I wasn't used to being on my own.

After the stroke I suffered epilepsy, which is a big thing. It gives you bad anxiety, especially if you are on your own. It's okay if you're in a house and a safe place. You sometimes have absent seizures, where you get twitches, which I get. I have petit mal seizures if I don't have enough sleep, drink too much, or don't have enough sugar in my system. They are controlled now, but it's scary. You have to be around people you know will understand. So when I go to Uni I ask the person, 'do you know what to do if I have a seizure? If not, look in my pocket and get this card out'.

A lot of people I thought I was close to, they say, 'what do I actually do if you have a seizure?' I just think I can't be around them and feel safe. So you shut yourself away from that person. I've learned not to use my stroke in a bad way now, but if someone said 'let's do this', and I've said 'I can't'. Obviously there are normal things like swimming or running I genuinely can't do because of it, but in terms of other things; like 'we'll go here', and I'm tired, I'll say, 'I can't, my stroke's really bad'. But that's probably the only time it's been an excuse.

It's difficult to think you'll ever be normal again, and people recover in different ways. I'd say to anyone else, keep thinking positively and keep reminding yourself you're still alive and with stroke you can get better. And they've treated it so your chances of having another one are probably low. Take yourself away from people who aren't true friends, and train your brain not to need them. And don't push yourself too much. So don't walk if you're tired, and don't overdo it.

I'm so different now - in a good way. Not so anxious. When I first had the stroke I used to look quite unapproachable. I didn't make any friends at Uni at first because I looked down at the floor and would hold my arms too tight. People thought I didn't want anyone in my life and needed to be alone.

I joined the gym through the summer, through Exercise Referral, which I wouldn't even have done before my stroke, which made my fatigue better. I'm more outgoing. I'm more approachable, so if people ask me if I'm okay, instead of just going 'yeah', I'm asking them and have conversations. I don't hold my arm as tight. I still protect it. I don't walk as slow and I just get on with my life. That's all you can do after a stroke, otherwise you won't recover, because your brain needs to know there is life after stroke.

If I can't do something; if I'm sitting at dinner and get really tired I'm always like 'oh it's my stroke, it's taking over'. If I'm walking downstairs and people are waiting behind me I make a joke, 'oh, there'll be a traffic jam, so go first.' It's things like that I get really embarrassed about. I think, I was never like this before my stroke and hate how I'm different. But other than that I'm not as depressed as I was.

I had another boyfriend after my stroke. It was an unhealthy relationship. I just wanted someone to love me. I wanted to be in a relationship so I'd seem like I was happy when I wasn't. He treated me badly, and took my vulnerability to a whole new level.

My new boyfriend, he didn't know me before my stroke so he accepts me. He says 'you are who you are and that's how I know you'. I think he saw the confidence coming out of me after the last ex dumped me. I was all depressed about it - on Facebook - and then suddenly I came out of my shell, and thought, 'I'm going back to Uni'. I was allowed to do that. I wasn't as vulnerable, so he just found me and we're really happy. We're engaged.

Going back to Uni I needed my brain to be in gear. It was difficult, but it kind of just came. It was sticking to routine, which is quite boring, reading a lot of my notes, just telling myself I needed to get my memory back. I still do stupid little things, like nearly leaving the front door open, but then remember to check it. It's never been that bad. But it's training the brain, just thinking and doing stuff.

I spend hours at the gym. If I think, I can't do it, I'm tired, I think, if I can spend an hour at the gym I can stay at Uni for longer - if I've done it before I can do it again. That's how I get through and motivated.

I call stroke the hidden injury because you can't see it. Your brain is such a big thing; it controls everything. You forget things; you're tired. People dismiss it. They think 'you can walk, you can do this, you're fine now, you're recovered.' They ask what percentage you think your recovery is. Everyone is different and I get angry when I see these articles - like Chris Tarrant, who was probably thrombolysed; caught in the four hour space - who says, like, 'I'm recovered now, I can do everything'. And then you look at Andrew Marr. Everyone is different.

The thing that annoys me most is when I'm really tired, and people say 'oh you're always tired, and you don't do anything'. When you're tired you just want to sit in and watch TV, eat food. Also the whole 'why do you put yourself down, you need to be confident and stronger, you were like that before your stroke'. You think to yourself, you get embarrassed and ashamed. But I'm past that now and I think 'I am who I am'.

I think it's for the best. You are a new person. You can almost start your life from fresh, obviously in an adult's body with a child's brain. But you can create who you want to be, and never got the chance to be. You find out who your friends are and you realise how much family means to you. A lot of people have said recently that I seem very mature. Being at Uni and in a relationship you have to be. And I think what I've been through, it's taught me to grow up properly.

AFTERWORD

Will Davison:

It intrigues me that I am exactly fifty years older that Lizzie Ashmore, but agree entirely with her sentiments. It's a fact that my two strokes have also done me a favour.

Earlier in my life I had worked at a TV producer, making regular weekly programmes for and about disabled people. I was used to pressure, or so I thought. But when that period of my life ended, I felt I needed a job that would give me something to do.

I was home alone; my wife Annie was in France visiting a friend. I got myself a part-time job as a kitchen assistant in a local village public house and was looking forward to being useful and earning again. I was sixty years old.

The night before I started work, I felt a little anxious. Later that evening I felt a small 'ping' in my right thigh. Nothing more. I went to bed.

The kitchen proved very stressful. Chef – and his assistant – kept me busy. It wasn't the easiest working atmosphere. One hour in I felt very strange. My right leg wasn't working properly. I realised I had begun limping badly, but I had no rational thought about what was happening to me. No doubt I was in shock. Perhaps if I'd witnessed it in someone else I could and would have done something. But my mind seemed cut off from what was happening to my body.

I had to get out of the kitchen. I told them I was feeling ill and somehow limped out. I managed to get into my car and drove home using my left foot on the gas pedal. It sounds like madness but I had to get home. That's where I needed to be. Somehow I coped with gears and accelerator – even crossing a major road.

As I walked in the cat ran away from me, scared of my staggering gait. I lay down and breathed a sign of relief. Eventually he came over and sat on my paralysed right leg. At some point – I don't know when or why – I put two potatoes on to bake. I was completely in denial of what was happening. I seriously thought, in time it would go away and I'll just get better!

Later a neighbour came to the back door. She insisted I go to the doctor's surgery, which was only three hundred yards away in the village. I leant on cottage walls to balance myself as I staggered down the pavement. At the surgery I was told to wait. I didn't say 'I'm really sick', and certainly not 'I'm having a stroke'. I had no idea how serious it was.

Twenty minutes later my GP told me what was happening and ordered an ambulance. He also told me to stay very calm and walk home carefully. Our neighbour kindly packed my bag upstairs and then I remembered the baked potatoes. She put them in foil and I went off in the ambulance. Why did I need them?

The paramedic sat me down and we drove ten miles to the local hospital. Facing backwards I felt sick and he produced a bowl. I wasn't sick, just scared.

I was politely checked in and given a bed in a spare room that was really a store. It's all a bit hazy now but I do clearly recall white-coated staff coming in, apologising, calling me 'sir', collecting supplies and leaving. Eventually a doctor came to see me, but the hospital obviously didn't have a spare bed, so I stayed put.

Later I felt hungry, starving in fact. There was nobody around and no food had been mentioned. So I opened my overnight bag and ate a baked potato. I gave huge thanks for baking it earlier in the day.

It was dark outside – I was still in my own clothes - when a nurse came to take me to a ward. I'd have to walk, she said. The porters had gone off duty and she wasn't allowed to push me in a wheelchair. I limped along what felt like miles of corridor and ended up parked in the corner of a ward. No curtain, but a bed at least. I managed to leave a message for my daughter who fortunately lived only a mile from the hospital.

I was asked by the man in the bed opposite what was wrong with me. My GP had said 'stroke', and that's what I told him. 'Oh I had one several years ago. You'll be walking again very soon. Don't worry.'

His words of encouragement bucked me up no end. It was an act of great generosity at exactly the right time. I can see why hospitals are unwilling to say such things, but at that moment I needed empathy and encouragement.

Sad to say, next day I heard a consultant tell the very same man that his condition, whatever it was, was fatal. He was going to die. The man's only – and very gentle – response was to ask the doctor to tell his family in private, not out loud in the open ward. That was twelve years ago and even the **'#Hello my name is'** campaign has taken all this time to get started. Hospitals can indeed be brutal, unfeeling places.

My elder daughter arrived the next morning, which was a great comfort to me; wonderfully followed by my brother and his wife. I was touched that my family had rallied round so quickly. After lunch Annie arrived. She had rushed back from France, full of concern. I was taken down for x-rays, ultrasound and an MRI scan. Later a consultant looked me over and read the scans.

I'd obviously lost some, hopefully small, part of my brain, but I was alive. A day later I was discharged.

Only weeks before I had raced down our street with my granddaughter. Against the odds I had beaten her and she said, 'Oh, you do run fast granddad!' That was the last time I ran for my life! I am now a walker, not a runner. And that saddens me.

Annie drove me home and I stayed in bed for three days. The cat came and lay beside my right leg for two days but after lunch on the third day he obviously considered me sufficiently healed and went off about his business.

The next day I got up and began the long slow process of walking myself back to normality – or as close as I could get to it. Our local Red Cross branch (it was still a time when they had local branches) loaned me a stick and I walked morning and afternoon. At first I managed twenty yards to a local tree; then fifty yards to the square. Each day a little further. Every time I came home and just lay down and slept. My right leg started to work a little better; less stiffness, a bit more mobility. But I was so weary!

I had been placed on blood pressure pills, statins, and aspirin to thin my blood, but I had such bad headaches I eventually went back to the consultant. She said 'I'm amazed you lasted that long. Most people manage a fortnight. They either work or they don't!' The new prescription sorted out the headaches and I began to feel much better.

My friend in the bed opposite was right. Several months later I was walking again moderately well, maybe with a limp, but I was fine. I had been allowed three sessions of physiotherapy and was told that if I missed one that would be it! The physio felt I was fine to get on with my life. So I continued exercising myself.

Six months later I was bored and volunteered to work abroad. I was to train a bright young charity worker to make videos in China. My GP advanced me six months medication.

On the plane I was so lucky to sit next to a man of about my own age who indicated he had Parkinson's disease. We talked a great deal and I realised my fear of my own post stroke adventure was nothing compared to his courage in setting out on a walking tour of China. It was apparent when he moved around the cabin just how physically difficult life had become for him. He said he was undertaking this trip as a final foray before the disease put him 'in lockup' as he called it. A very brave man who gave me courage.

Annie and I lived in Beijing for six months. Annie took up mandarin classes and Handicap International showed me a China I could never have seen as a tourist. I loved the filming in China and especially Tibet.

The greatest joy was riding to work in Lhasa on the back of my HI interpreter's motorbike, passing the Potala Palace, going to Tibet's Television Centre. I felt absolutely in heaven!

However my blood pressure pills increasingly caused reactions: swelling and pain in my lower limbs, and an intensely itchy skin. I had no means of changing the prescription until I returned to the UK. To counter the pain in my legs I regularly walked home from the HI Beijing office every day under the fifth ring road.

On my return to the UK, I changed medication, my GP telling me it was a question of finding the right drug for me. They all have side effects! It's the one that suits you best.

Five years on, itchy feet again caused Annie and I to move on to France where we renovated an old farmhouse in Normandy. One Saturday I went to a nearby town to order a patio door to replace the leaky original. I met Steve, our builder friend, and we sorted out the order. I knew I felt very anxious – uncomfortable, perhaps, and a bit 'not there'. Steve looked worried and said, 'are you okay? You look ill. Are you going to die on me?'

I did feel increasingly odd. There was no physical manifestation, but I did feel deeply anxious. Once again I drove home. At no point did I think 'I'm having another stroke'. I made a cup of tea in the kitchen, sat down and tried to relax. Annie was out swimming. I decided to go to bed. I would feel better after a sleep.

I managed the stairs, but the decision to have tea and go upstairs was a bad one, as I later discovered. When Annie got home she immediately took charge and called the Sapeurs Pompier (who carry out fire and ambulance duties in France). In hindsight I realise Annie must have thought through the possibility of another stroke as she had listed all the necessary numbers in case of an emergency.

Four big lads arrived. It's strange when you are the object being rescued nobody speaks to you. Maybe it was the language barrier. They called a second crew as our stairs were too difficult to carry me down and they didn't want me to walk. I insisted on going to the loo and then they strapped me onto a stretcher and manoeuvred me down the staircase. It's a scene I've played through in my head many times since – I could have been in a box!

The journey to hospital took twenty-five minutes along the autoroute. I became so desperate to pee, and the only advantage to that was it distracted me from what was happening. Male pride: I wasn't going to wet myself!

Annie followed by car and we met up in casualty where I was put on a trolley in the emergency room. Thankfully I was given a bottle to pee. That was okay the first time, but it got worse. I was soon desperate to pee again, I reached for a distant bottle and fell off the trolley, landed on the floor unable to move, and worse still revealing my bare backside to the world. Hospital gowns are very revealing! Annie and the nurse heard me shout and rushed in to rescue me. I felt embarrassed at the time, but now see the funny side of that stroke experience.

Soon after I had an X-ray, and a couple of hours later was taken by wheelchair to a surgical ward (they too were short of beds) and shared a room with a gentleman recovering from surgery.

In bed I began assiduously exercising my foot. I had paralysis in my right leg. The next morning I was given a typical French breakfast. And I was starving. The nurses were charming and very kind and with supervision I got out of bed to have a shower. I quickly realised I had more impairment from this stroke than the previous one. My right leg was much stiffer, as was my right hand.

Daily I exercised my hand bending and stretching my fingers. I also became aware my memory was problematic, so I went over and over the names of my seven grandchildren as an exercise. My speech was affected and I was finding more difficult to say some words. On Monday morning I was transferred to a medical ward and put into a side room where I could watch the traffic on the autoroute. I did feel trapped!

I was wheeled down for tests and was reassured that the ultrasound on my neck appeared to be okay. The radiologist told me in excellent English that all appeared to be well. Then I was taken to the MRI chamber. The French scanner was an early model and tiny compared to the one in Swindon. It was told it would last twenty minutes.

Despite being given an alarm button I felt so closed in – I'd never experienced claustrophobia like this. I decided to try self-hypnosis in an attempt to calm myself down. I counted backwards slowly. Months later, my builder friend Steve told me he kept a Valium tablet in his wallet just in case he had to go through that same scanner again!

Given the damage caused by the stroke, the MRI was apparently satisfactory, but I was kept in for the week to ensure I was stable. One of the joys of the French hospital system is that we had two senior doctors permanently on our ward. They would do medical rounds every morning but remain on the ward all day. France is more informal – so if you want to talk to the doctors they are readily accessible – and very chatty.

At the end of the week I was able to limp around and went down to the window alcove at the end of the corridor. Both doctors sat with Annie and me and showed us the X-ray where we could see the tiny hole in my brain, the result of the stroke. We chatted about my situation. I asked could I do some gardening? Could I cut the grass? Will my speech improve?

The answers were simple: take time, go steady; allow improvements to take shape in their own time. I told them I wanted to go home and they discharged me into the care of my wife. I was so relieved! Again Annie proved a lifesaver. She was so positive and always encouraged me to see myself as getting stronger and better.

Once more I began working on my stiff right leg - and this time round my poor diction. Strangely I found that before I uttered certain words I knew they wouldn't come out right. I could tell people had difficulty understanding me and it was intensely frustrating. Our neighbour Maurice couldn't cope, I spoke to him every day and I could see he found my speech such a difficulty for him and would turn away to Annie to respond.

The second stroke was more troublesome than the first. It took much more effort to get myself back to 'normal' You don't realise what normal is until you loose it. I still felt out of place and my balance had deteriorated. With Annie's help we decided to plant some beans in our veg patch. I couldn't easily get down on my knees but when I did and eventually got up, I stumbled and fell headlong backwards into the raspberry canes. We both laughed - and got the message that this was not going to be a quick fix.

Again I started walking every day. The same routine: this time along the lane leading to our house - one telephone pole; two telephone poles, until I could get to the main road. If I dawdled, or chatted to a neighbour, Annie would appear at the gate looking for me, or I would get a text saying, 'U Ok?' I always carried my mobile, just in case.

Every morning I sat in bed for an hour or so, writing by hand. I wrote hundreds of individual letters of the alphabet every day. At first my scrawl was just that, a scrawl. But later my longhand steadied and although it wasn't brilliant it was legible. More importantly I felt much better about it.

I did find it difficult to say certain words. Elisabeth – a friend in France – I had to refer to as Lizzie. S or sss were difficult, and I soon realised that mentally I changed what I was going to say because I knew in advance I wouldn't be able to say a particular word. It was like a stream of words that had a log jam in it. Paraphrasing was the answer.

I found communication problems irritating and frustrating. Awareness of the problem added to the difficulty. People had problems understanding me, which in itself silenced me. It had become a confidence issue.

An early edition of QI (BBC TV) featured Nina Conti, the ventriloquist, who talked about the art of using the stomach to produce speech without lip movement. 'Venting' definitely works, and with practise you can talk clearly using the solar plexus. Using your tummy as a sounding board gives projection and power to speech and the more I tried this over the next months, the clearer my speech became, and my confidence grew.

In the early stages it was really helpful to have such positive feedback from Annie who encouraged me to exercise and speak. I only reverted to 'stroke speech', as I called it, when I was stressed or nervous. But even now if I'm in a group of strangers or at a party Annie says I am more hesitant in speech than I need be. It doesn't happen when we are just the two of us. In more recent times, attending Stroke Club has definitely given me the confidence to speak out more.

There was also the added difficulty of what I discovered on the internet is called 'slow thinking' where memories and thoughts take time to reach the foreground of the mind. I assumed that a re-wiring of my brain was in progress and that it would take time to settle down. So it proved. It still takes time to remember – but I know it's there somewhere! Just give it time.

Most people were polite enough not to mention it, but when I was walking in our local town I noticed I limped more – for being seen in public. One of the most difficult things for me was attending a nephew's wedding and revealing for the first time to my family that I had a physical impairment. 'Coming out' in stroke terms.

There were times when I felt trapped in my body – a not quite fit for purpose body, but somehow I managed to leave any depression behind by taking time alone. I had a routine when I felt depressed, I would isolate myself – rather than spread the negativity around – drink mugs of tea and realise I was so lucky to be alive.

On the plus side, it dawned on me that I had had a change of personality. My quick fire temper that would jump out alarmingly, causing me (and those around me) great surprise and embarrassment – and upset – had gone. It was amazing to realise I no longer found life so challenging. I now had a much calmer worldview.

My temper has gone; burnt out in the fire of a stroke. I don't understand the mechanism but I know the end result. Wonderful. The drive, and presumably the anger, that had motivated me to create things had been moderated into a quieter, calmer way of being. There is certainly less drama now.

Life is perhaps more gentle and easier to live – for me and for everyone else.

Twelve years since the beginning of this adventure, I am able to do things more or less as before. My right leg feels different, heavier, less flexible, but, with a stick to aid my poor balance, to all intents and purposes it works. (And it was only when I started using a stick that I realised how many other people needed to use one). I can't walk as far, or for that long. I do get so tired and have to rest.

I can't do what I did pre-stroke, but then I am older now. It's a quieter less stressful life and really all the better for that. Who wouldn't yearn for the vigour of their early years; but not the anxiety. I'm afraid I'll have to leave all that excitement to the grandchildren.

One thing I have learned from the recent interviews I've conducted for this book. Everybody who has had a stroke has had to face the loss of their old self: the running, jumping version of themselves, and face up to a newly emerged reality.

It can be painful but the new you is the real you. And you are alive. It is just so vital to make the most of the life you've got.

ACKNOWLEDGEMENTS

Special thanks to Bill Stammers of Stroke Club UK; Lorraine Ayres and Dave Cottrell of Different Strokes; and Anil Ranchod and Daisy Dighton of the Stroke Association, for introducing me to potential interviewees.

Jo Harrison for collating the book and Ryan Ashcroft of Love Your Covers for his cover design.

Cover photographs of stroke survivor contributors by Will Davison. Brendan Kehoe photograph by Sue Ballard. Author photograph by Annie Davison.

For further information on **'So You've Had a Stroke'** go to:

www.willdavison.info

Printed in Great Britain
by Amazon